Top 100 Finger Foods

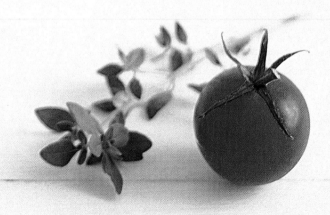

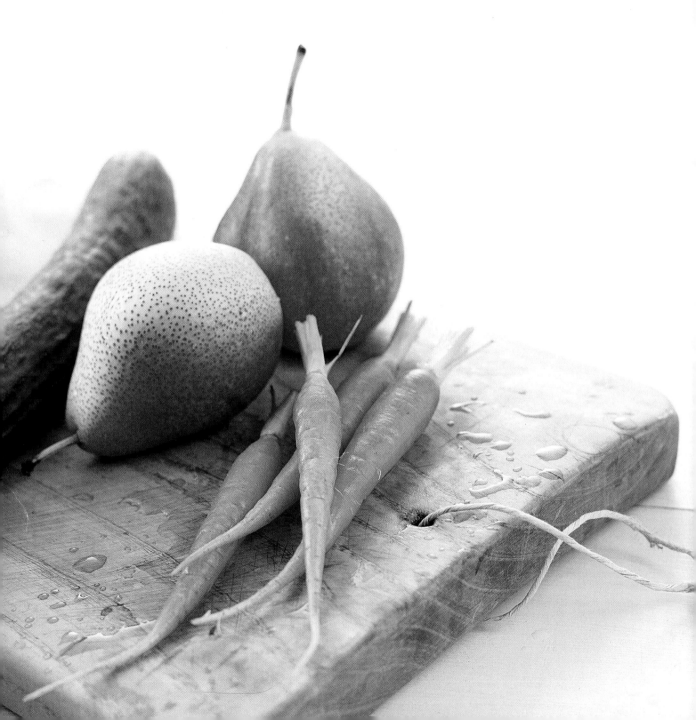

Annabel Karmel
Top 100 Finger Foods

100 recipes for a healthy, happy child

ATRIA BOOKS

New York   London   Toronto   Sydney

For my children, Nicholas, Lara, and Scarlett, and Oscar, my puppy, who gets to enjoy the leftovers

ATRIA BOOKS
A Division of Simon & Schuster, Inc.
1230 Avenue of the Americas
New York, NY 10020

First Atria Books hardcover edition February 2010

ATRIA BOOKS and colophon are trademarks of Simon & Schuster, Inc.

For information about special discounts for bulk purchases, please contact Simon & Schuster Special Sales at 1-866-506-1949 or business@simonandschuster.com.

The Simon & Schuster Speakers Bureau can bring authors to your live event. For more information or to book an event, contact the Simon & Schuster Speakers Bureau at 1-866-248-3049 or visit our website at www.simonspeakers.com.

Manufactured in the United States of America

10   9   8   7   6   5   4   3   2   1

Library of Congress Cataloging-in-Publication Data
Karmel, Annabel.
   Top 100 finger foods : 100 recipes for a healthy, happy child / Annabel Karmel.
      p.   cm.
   Includes index.
   1. Cookery (Baby foods)   2. Infants—Nutrition.   I. Title.
   TX740.K294   2009
   641.5'6222—dc22   2009038972

ISBN 978-0-7434-9371-0
ISBN 978-1-4391-6495-2 (ebook)

Please note that all flour is all-purpose unless otherwise specified, all butter is unsalted, milk is whole milk, and eggs are large. Flour measures are spooned and leveled.

Contents

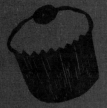

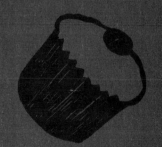

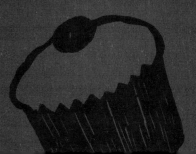

Introduction

First Finger Foods

Until now, feeding your baby has been your job, but at around 8 or 9 months old, your little one will start to want to do this on his own. Quite often, babies are determined to feed themselves before they have the level of coordination required to use a spoon. This is an age when children experiment with their food, and if you are the type of person who likes everything neat and tidy, you are going to have to draw a deep breath, as your child will want to play with his or her food. Children are going to want to touch, hold, drop, and, occasionally, throw their food.

Finger foods are about to become an increasingly important part of your baby's diet, and the more you allow your child to experiment, the more quickly he will learn to feed himself. Don't be concerned if your child ends up wearing most of his food. At this early stage, it's simply practice. But do keep offering finger foods and more lumpy textures, as these will help refine your baby's chewing technique, which in turn helps with speech development and strengthens your baby's jaw muscles. Interestingly, many babies refuse to eat lumpy food from a spoon or fork but will eat finger foods even though these also require chewing.

Good first finger foods

Initially, it's important to choose foods that are quite soft, as babies can bite off a piece of a hard food like raw carrot and choke on it—so to start off, I like to offer the following:

- Steamed vegetables such as carrot or sweet potato sticks, small broccoli or cauliflower florets
- Soft ripe fruit: for example, banana, peach, melon, mango
- Sticks of toast or broiled cheese toast
- Cooked pasta shapes with a very small amount of sauce or a little melted butter and grated cheese

Finger foods for older babies

Among the suggestions that follow, there are lots of accompanying recipes throughout the book from which to choose.

- Sticks of cheese
- Raw vegetables, such as carrot and cucumber sticks
- Apple slices, strawberries, blueberries, halved or quartered peeled grapes
- Dried fruits, such as apricots and apples—try to use the soft type and avoid California apricots, which are very tart.
- Unsweetened breakfast cereals
- Rice cakes
- Mini meatballs or burgers
- Pieces of chicken or fish with or without a crumb coating
- Cold cuts, sliced wafer-thin and rolled up into a cigar shape

- Pita bread, flatbreads, bagels
- Mini sandwiches—mashed banana, cream cheese, peanut butter (Provided there is no history of allergy or atopic disease in your family—for example, hay fever, asthma, or eczema—it should be fine to give peanut butter from 7 months on.)
- Mini homemade pizzas
- Mini muffins
- Mini homemade cookies
- Mini ice pops made from fresh fruit

Checklist for First Finger Foods

1 Peel apples and pears initially, but as your baby gets older, introduce the skin as well, as the vitamins lie just below it.

2 Often it's better to give a large piece of fruit or vegetable that your child can hold and eat rather than bite-size pieces.

3 When making sandwiches for little ones, it's a good idea to slightly flatten the bread first with a rolling pin so that the sandwich is not too thick for your child to eat.

4 There is no need to be obsessive about germs. It's fine to use an antibacterial wipe to clean your baby's high chair—but remember that your baby picks things up from the floor and puts them in her mouth all the time.

5 Your baby's hands should always be washed before she eats.

6 One very common thing that pediatric dieticians talk about is children who are afraid of mess. This seems to be at the root of many toddler eating problems. Allow your baby to experiment—she's bound to get into a mess, but it's not a good idea to continually wipe your child's face clean while she is eating.

7 Try not to buy dried apricots that are treated with sulfur dioxide to preserve their bright orange color, as this can trigger an asthma attack in susceptible babies.

8 A large mat placed under the high chair to catch food and recycle it is a good investment.

Choking

Just because your child can chew off a piece of food, like a chunk of raw carrot or apple, doesn't mean that she can swallow it down properly. Sometimes children bite off pieces of food and then store them in their mouth, so always check when your child comes out of the high chair that there is no lumpy food left in her mouth.

Foods that are choking hazards include:
- Pieces of raw vegetables
- Grapes—you should peel grapes and cut them in half or into quarters
- Raisins
- Fruit with pits
- Cherry or grape tomatoes—best to quarter these
- Chunks of hard cheese
- Nuts

What to do if your child chokes:
- If your child chokes, check inside his mouth and remove any object, but be careful not to push the object farther down his throat.
- Lay your baby facedown on your forearm with his head lower than his chest. Give him five sharp slaps on the middle of his back with your other hand.
- If this does not dislodge the object, turn your baby over onto his back and, pushing down with two fingers in the middle of his chest, make five sharp thrusts at a rate of about one every 3 seconds. Then check your baby's mouth again for any obstruction.
- If unsuccessful, call 911 immediately.

Teething

Some babies are born with teeth, some get them at 6 months old, and some may have hardly any teeth by the time they are 1 year old. While some babies sail through teething, it can be a pretty miserable time for others. Telltale teething signs include bright red cheeks, inflamed gums, mild rash around the mouth, mild fever, irritability, and changes in feeding and sleeping patterns. As a parent, I believe it's very important to trust your

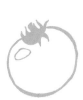

instincts, and you know better than anyone when something is not right with your baby. There is divided opinion among experts on whether teething can cause a mild fever or diarrhea. However, they all agree that you should check with your doctor if you are concerned about your baby, and don't just put it down to teething.

Some ways to help your baby:

While babies are teething, it is not unusual for them to be off their food. It is a good idea to keep some chilled cucumber sticks in the fridge, put banana in the freezer, or make some fresh fruit ice pops. Cold foods help to soothe sore gums. You can also dampen some clean washcloths, freeze them, and then offer them to your child to chew on.

Offer your child some cool, smooth foods like applesauce or yogurt.

Gel-filled teething rings that can be put in the fridge can also help cool sore gums.

You can rub sugar-free teething gel on your baby's gums or give some infants' Tylenol if your baby has a slight fever, but always check with your pediatrician before giving any medication to your baby.

If your baby uses a pacifier, then keep a supply of chilled pacifiers in the fridge.

Cuddle or nurse your baby—a baby feels less uncomfortable if relaxed and happy. Try to distract her by offering a change in scenery, a new toy, or a fun activity—this will make it harder for her to concentrate on being miserable.

Rub petroleum jelly around the outside of your baby's mouth to protect it from becoming red and sore when your baby dribbles.

Make sure that you brush your child's teeth as soon as they appear. Use a baby toothbrush and a smear of infant toothpaste.

Try to avoid soda and other sugary beverages. Give only milk or water in a bottle. However, you can give juice at mealtimes in a sippy cup, but make sure it has no added sugar. It is best to restrict juice to mealtimes, when there is plenty of saliva in the mouth to wash away the acid.

Breakfast Bites

A good breakfast should contain protein such as eggs, cheese, or yogurt; whole-grain cereal or bread; and some fresh fruit. Your idea of breakfast is bound to be different from your child's. Be flexible—my children have been known to eat odd things for breakfast like toasted English muffins spread with tomato sauce and topped with tomatoes and grated Cheddar, then popped under the broiler. If there's a rush in the morning and no time to sit and eat breakfast, give your child a healthy fruit muffin and a smoothie to take with him on his journey.

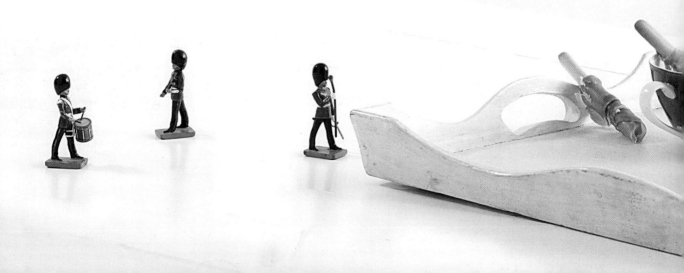

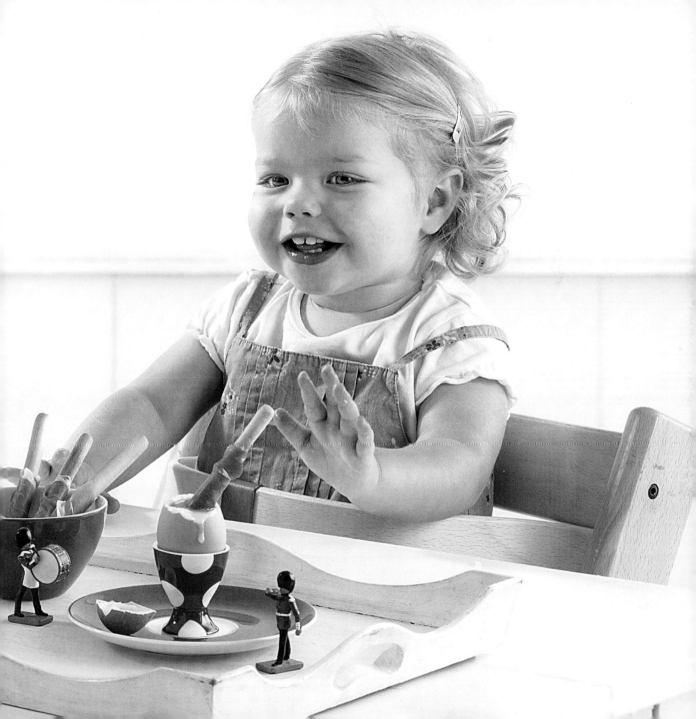

Fluffy Finger-Sized Pancakes

🥞 Preparation 7 minutes
🕐 Cook 20 minutes (assuming 5 batches)
🍳 Makes about 24 small or 8 large pancakes, 4 to 6 portions
☺ Suitable for children under 1
❄ Suitable for freezing

1/2 cup self-rising flour
1 tablespoon sugar
1/4 teaspoon baking soda
a pinch of salt (optional)
1 egg
3 tablespoons milk
1 tablespoon vegetable oil, for frying
1/4 cup plain or vanilla yogurt
2 teaspoons maple syrup

Pancakes are yummy for breakfast and also make a nice dessert for both kids and adults. Try them with fruits such as sliced bananas, strawberries, or blueberries, too.

Whisk the flour, sugar, baking soda, and salt, if using, together in a medium bowl. Beat the egg and milk together in a separate bowl and add to the dry ingredients, then mix together until just combined. Let the batter stand for 5 minutes—it will thicken slightly, and you will see some bubbles forming.

Meanwhile, heat a large, heavy-bottomed frying pan over medium heat. Brush a little of the oil on the bottom and drop teaspoonfuls of the batter into the pan. For larger pancakes, use tablespoonfuls of batter. Cook for 1 1/2 to 2 minutes, until the pancakes are golden on the bottom and bubbles have formed on the surface. Flip the pancakes over and cook for 1 to 2 minutes more, until they are cooked through and brown on the second side. Lower the heat slightly if they are browning too quickly.

Transfer the cooked pancakes to a plate and keep warm in a low oven. Re-oil the pan and continue cooking batches of pancakes until all of the batter has been used up.

Divide the yogurt among four small bowls and drizzle half a teaspoon of maple syrup over the top of each. Serve with the warm pancakes.

Suitable for freezing: Let the cooked pancakes cool, and wrap in foil. Reheat directly from frozen in an oven preheated to 400°F. Put the foil package(s) on a baking sheet and bake for 5 to 6 minutes. Let cool slightly before serving.

Breakfast Burrito

A burrito generally describes a filling completely enclosed by a flour tortilla or wrap. It gets its name from Mexico, where it was a popular "packed lunch" for traveling (*burro* is Spanish for donkey). But nowadays burritos are popular everywhere, especially for breakfast. For a mild salsa recipe, see Nachos (page 27), or use your favorite store-bought one.

Whisk the egg and milk together in a small bowl and season to taste with salt and pepper. Melt the butter in a small frying pan and add the egg mixture. Cook gently, stirring, until the egg is softly scrambled.

Warm the tortilla for 10 to 15 seconds in a microwave or for 1 minute in a dry frying pan. Spoon the scrambled egg down the center of the tortilla (not quite to the edges at the top and bottom), and add the salsa and cheese. Fold the top and bottom of the tortilla inward, then roll the wrap up from the left-hand side so that the filling is completely enclosed. Serve immediately.

Preparation 5 minutes
Cook 5 minutes
Makes 1 portion
Not suitable for freezing or reheating

1 egg
1 tablespoon milk or cream
salt and pepper, to season
a pat of butter
one 7-inch flour tortilla
1 tablespoon mild salsa or
 ½ tomato, seeded and diced
1 heaping tablespoon grated
 Cheddar

Optional add-ins
You can add variety by including extra fillings to the basic recipe. Some of my favorites are:

1 slice bacon, cooked until
 crisp, then crumbled
1 cooked new potato, diced
 and sautéed in a little oil
 until golden
1 small slice ham, cut into cubes
 or small strips
1 tablespoon drained canned
 corn, added to the egg so
 that it heats through
2 or 3 mushrooms, thinly sliced
 and sautéed in a little oil

Soft-Boiled Egg with "Italian Soldiers"

Preparation 5 minutes
Cook 4 minutes
Makes 1 portion (easily increased)

1 egg
2 breadsticks (grissini)
2 slices prosciutto or Parma ham

My new twist on a British nursery favorite of eggs and soldiers (toast sticks). I like to vary this sometimes by using sesame-coated breadsticks. The "Italian soldiers" would also make a nice change for a lunch box, in double the quantity. Do not, though, give lightly cooked eggs to babies under the age of one.

Put a large saucepan of water over high heat and bring to a boil, then reduce the heat slightly to a brisk simmer. Gently lower in the egg using a spoon, and cook the egg for 4 minutes (for a runny yolk and a set white).

Meanwhile, break the breadsticks in half and cut the slices of prosciutto in half lengthwise. Wrap one of the pieces of prosciutto around one of the breadstick halves, starting at the broken end, and wrap twisting downward and slightly overlapping, so that around two-thirds of the breadstick is wrapped in ham. Press the ham firmly on itself to seal. Repeat so that you have four "Italian soldiers."

Transfer the egg to an egg cup and cut off the top. Dip the Italian soldiers in the egg yolk and enjoy!

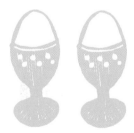

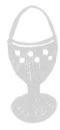

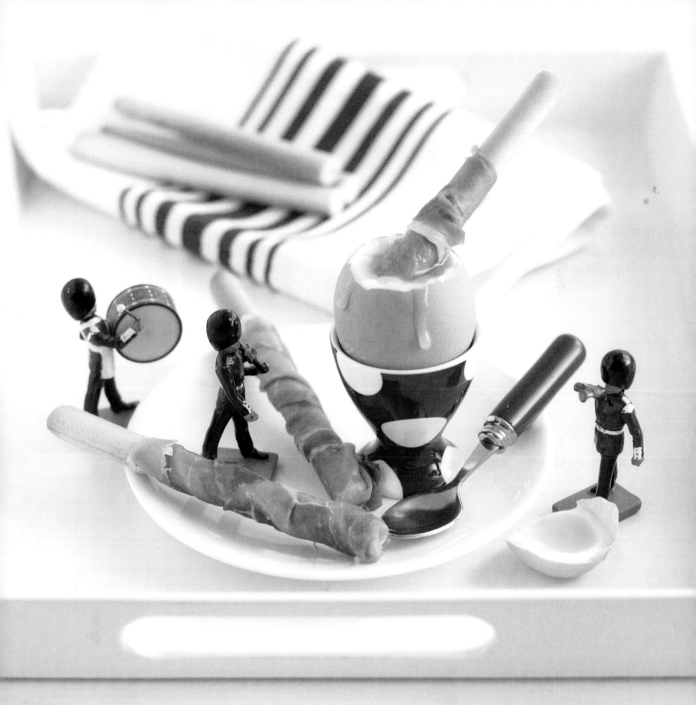

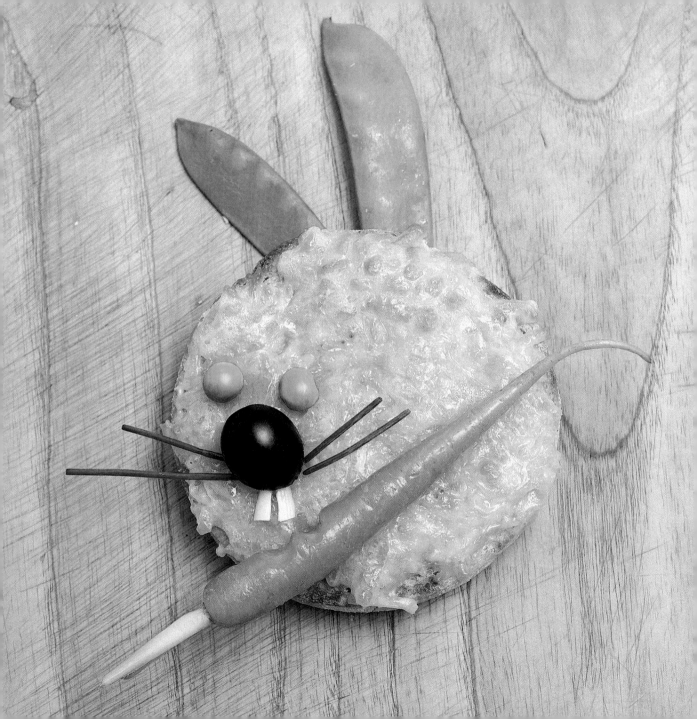

Welsh "Rabbits"

Welsh rarebit is a slightly enriched version of cheese toast—children will probably enjoy this version of "rabbit."

Preheat the broiler to high. Put the cheese, egg yolk, cream, and Worcestershire sauce into a bowl and mash together. Season to taste with pepper. Spread the cheese mixture on the cut sides of the toasted muffin, spreading right to the edges. Place the cheese-topped muffin halves about 3 inches away from the heat source (one rack down from normal broiling position)—don't have them too close, as the egg in the mixture can make them brown very quickly. Broil for 3 to 4 minutes, until the cheese has melted and is golden and bubbling.

Decorate the cooked muffin halves with peas for eyes and strips of carrot or snow peas for ears, half an olive for a nose, chives for whiskers, and scallion for teeth. Serve immediately.

🍳 Preparation 5 minutes
🕐 Cook 4 minutes
🥧 Makes 1 portion
❄ Not suitable for freezing or reheating

¹/₃ cup grated Cheddar
1 egg yolk
1 teaspoon cream or milk
2 or 3 drops Worcestershire sauce (or to taste)
pepper, to season
1 English muffin, split and lightly toasted
peas, thin slices of carrot or snow peas, 1 black olive (pitted and halved), a few fresh chives, and scallion, to garnish

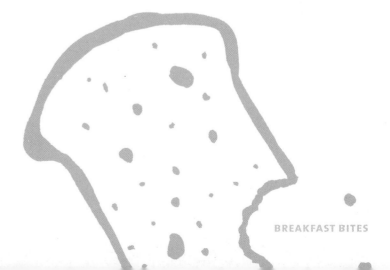

French Toast Sticks

🥣 Preparation 7 minutes
🕑 Cook 6 minutes
🍽 Makes 1 or 2 portions,
depending on age and appetite
☺ Suitable for children under 1
❄ Not suitable for freezing
or reheating

**2 slices white bread
1 tablespoon strawberry or
    raspberry jam
1 tablespoon reduced-fat
    cream cheese or Neufchâtel
    (optional)
1 egg
1 tablespoon cream or milk
1/2 teaspoon sugar
2 drops vanilla extract
1 tablespoon butter, for frying**

I like to use white bread, but feel free to use whole-grain. You can buy some very good sugar-free jam.

Roll the bread with a rolling pin to about half its original thickness and spread one slice with the jam. Spread the second slice with the cream cheese, if using, and sandwich together. Trim off the crusts, if you like. Beat the egg, cream, sugar, and vanilla together in a shallow dish.

Melt the butter in a frying pan over medium heat. Dip the jam sandwich into the egg mixture and turn over to coat. Put the egg-coated sandwich into the pan and fry for 2 to 3 minutes, until the underside is golden. Flip the sandwich over and cook for 2 to 3 minutes more, then transfer to a plate and carefully cut into sticks (a small serrated knife is good for this).

Allow to cool slightly and check the temperature before serving—be careful, as the jam can become very hot.

Mini Banana-Bran Muffins

🥣 Preparation 10 minutes
🕑 Cook 14 minutes
🍽 Makes 24 muffins
☺ Suitable for children under 1
❄ Suitable for freezing. Not
suitable for reheating.

**1 1/2 cups raisin bran flakes
5 tablespoons warm milk
1 medium banana, mashed
1 egg yolk**

There always seems to be the odd brown banana lurking in the bottom of the fruit bowl, and this is a great way to use it up. These are wonderful warm for breakfast or for an after-school snack.

Preheat the oven to 350°F. Line two 12-hole mini muffin pans with 24 paper cases.

Mix together the raisin bran flakes, milk, and banana, and let stand for 5 minutes. Transfer to a food processor with the egg yolk, oil, raisins, and sugar. Whiz for a minute to combine.

Add the flour, baking soda, baking powder, salt, cinnamon, and ginger, and pulse to combine. Spoon into the muffin cups (about 1 tablespoon for each mini muffin). Bake for 12 to 14 minutes, until risen and firm to the touch. Remove from the oven and allow to cool for 5 minutes, then transfer to a wire rack to cool completely.

Suitable for freezing: Baked muffins are best stored frozen. Freeze in a resealable container or freezer bag. Thaw for around 30 minutes at room temperature.

3 tablespoons canola oil
2 tablespoons raisins
1/3 cup (packed) light brown sugar
1/2 cup whole wheat flour
1/2 teaspoon baking soda
1/2 teaspoon baking powder
a generous pinch of salt
1/2 teaspoon ground cinnamon
1/4 teaspoon ground ginger

French Toast with Caramelized Bananas

Mix together the cream, milk, eggs, and vanilla. Cut the bread into triangles or sticks and put into a small, flat dish. Pour the egg mixture on top and let stand for 5 minutes, turning the bread over halfway through soaking.

Heat the pat of butter in a frying pan and allow to melt. Put the bread in the pan and fry gently over low heat for about 5 minutes on each side, until lightly golden.

Fry the bananas: Melt the butter in a small frying pan. Add the sugar. Add the bananas and fry gently until caramelized. Let the bananas cool slightly before serving, as caramelized sugar can get very hot. Serve the French toast with the bananas and sprinkle with a little sugar.

Preparation 12 minutes
Cook 10 minutes
Makes 2 portions
Suitable for children under 1
Not suitable for freezing or reheating

1/4 cup heavy cream
3 tablespoons milk
2 eggs
2 or 3 drops vanilla extract
1 thick slice white bread, preferably from an unsliced loaf
a pat of butter, for frying

For the caramelized bananas
1/2 tablespoon butter
1 tablespoon sugar
2 bananas, cut into thick slices at an angle
sugar, to sprinkle

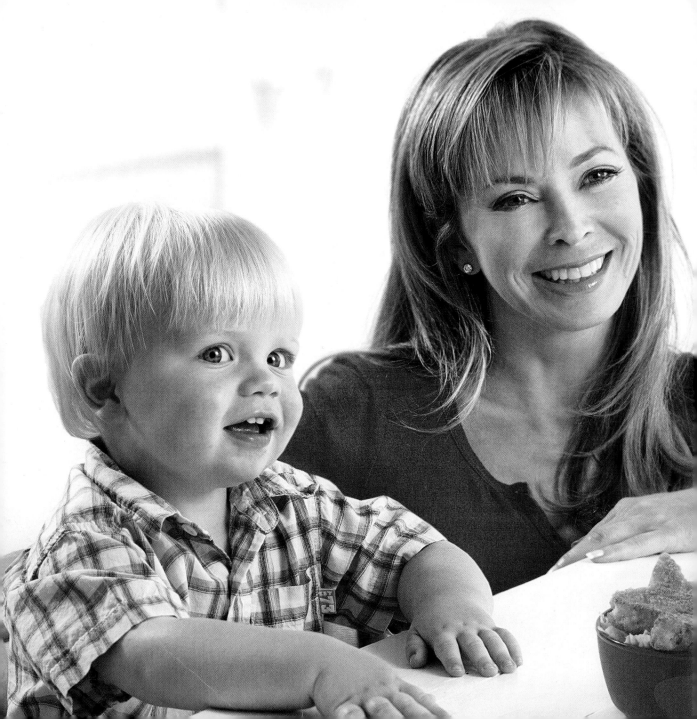

Versatile Veggies

Children need proportionally more fat than do adults, so for them a vegetarian diet should include foods such as cheese and eggs as well as avocados, nut butters, and seeds. Lack of iron is the most common deficiency in vegetarian children, so be sure to give iron-rich green leafy vegetables, egg yolks, fortified breakfast cereals, and dried fruit, especially apricots. Vitamin C–rich foods or a glass of orange juice with a meal helps boost iron absorption.

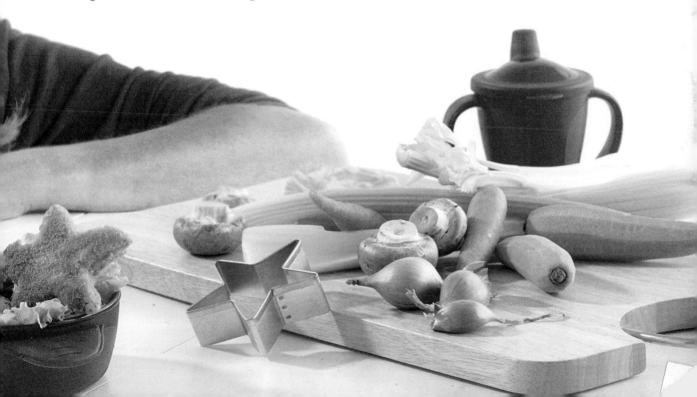

Carrot and Cheese Muffins

🍲 Preparation 15 minutes
🕐 Cook 16 minutes (mini)/
30 minutes (regular)
🍪 Makes 18 mini or 6 regular
muffins
❄ Suitable for freezing: Baked
muffins can be frozen in a
resealable container or freezer
bag. Thaw for 30 to 45 minutes
at room temperature. Not
suitable for reheating.

3/4 cup self-rising flour
1/4 teaspoon baking soda
a pinch of salt
a pinch of paprika
1/3 cup grated Cheddar
1/3 cup freshly grated Parmesan,
   plus 2 tablespoons extra
   for topping
2 tablespoons milk
2 tablespoons canola oil
1/4 cup plain yogurt
1 tablespoon maple syrup
1 egg
1 medium carrot, finely grated
1 teaspoon snipped fresh chives
   (optional)

Carrot is good in sweet muffins but equally nice in savory ones, too. It is a good way to hide a few extra vegetables to help you get your children to eat their healthy 5-a-day.

Preheat the oven to 350°F. Line mini muffin pans with 18 paper cases or a standard muffin pan with 6 paper cases.

Whisk the flour, baking soda, salt, paprika, and cheeses together in a bowl. Beat the milk, oil, yogurt, maple syrup, and egg together and stir into the dry ingredients, followed by the carrot and chives, if using. Drop heaping teaspoonfuls into the prepared muffin pan(s) (fill cups almost to the top). Sprinkle with the extra Parmesan and bake for 14 to 16 minutes for mini muffins, 25 to 30 minutes for regular-size muffins, until risen and golden brown.

Remove from the oven and allow to cool for 5 minutes, then transfer to a wire rack to cool completely.

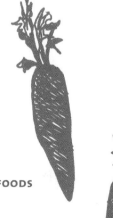

Cheese and Corn Muffins

Savory muffins are a slight change but all the better for it.
I like to serve these as a midmorning snack or breakfast
or, for older children, with soup for lunch.

Preheat the oven to 350°F. Line two 12-hole mini muffin
pans with 24 paper cases.

Put the corn and scallions in a food processor and whiz
until chopped. Add the yogurt, butter, honey, and egg, and whiz
to combine. Sift together the flour, baking soda, baking powder,
salt, and paprika, add to the yogurt mixture together with the
grated cheese, and pulse two or three times.

Spoon into the muffin cups (about three-quarters of a
tablespoon per cup). Bake for 12 to 14 minutes, until risen
and firm to the touch. Allow to cool in the pan for a few
minutes, then transfer to a wire rack to cool completely.

Preparation 10 minutes
Cook 14 minutes
Makes 24 muffins
Suitable for freezing:
Baked muffins can be frozen in
a resealable container or freezer
bag. Thaw for 30 to 45 minutes at
room temperature. Not suitable
for reheating.

½ cup drained canned corn
3 scallions, roughly sliced
¼ cup Greek-style yogurt
2 tablespoons butter, melted
  and cooled
1 tablespoon honey or maple
  syrup
1 egg
¾ cup flour or ½ cup flour
  and 2 tablespoons cornmeal
½ teaspoon baking soda
½ teaspoon baking powder
¼ teaspoon salt
⅛ teaspoon paprika
½ cup grated sharp Cheddar

Veggie Bites/Burgers

🍳 Preparation 20 minutes
🕐 Cook 16 minutes
🌀 Makes about 16 small bites
or 8 burgers
☺ Suitable for children under 1
❄ Suitable for freezing: Freeze
uncooked bites/burgers on baking
sheets lined with parchment paper.
When firm, transfer to freezer bags.
Cook directly from frozen, adding
1 minute extra cooking time for bites
and 2 minutes extra for burgers.

2 tablespoons olive oil
1 medium shallot, diced
½ celery stalk, diced
1 large carrot, peeled and grated
½ small leek, thinly sliced
3 cremini mushrooms, diced
1 garlic clove, crushed
1 tablespoon soy sauce
2 teaspoons light brown sugar
¼ cup freshly grated Parmesan
⅔ cup fresh bread crumbs
1½ teaspoons mayonnaise
1 heaping tablespoon grated Cheddar
salt and pepper, to season
5 tablespoons unseasoned dried
   bread crumbs
2 tablespoons flour
1 egg
2 to 3 tablespoons canola oil, for
   frying
buns, lettuce, tomato, mayonnaise,
   to serve (for burgers)

Ever met a vegetable-hating vegetarian? Well, I have met quite a few. These tasty veggie bites or burgers are a good way to encourage children to eat more vegetables, as here the veggies are mashed up—and not being visible, they can't be picked out.

Heat the olive oil in a large nonstick frying pan and sauté all the vegetables except the garlic for 10 minutes, or until soft. Add the garlic and cook for a minute, then add the soy sauce and sugar, and cook for 1 minute more. Spread out on a plate and let cool.

For small veggie bites, you need to chop the cooked and cooled veggies, either in a food processor (scraping down the sides frequently) or with a large knife.

Transfer the vegetables to a bowl and mix in 2 tablespoons of the Parmesan, the fresh bread crumbs, mayonnaise, Cheddar, and pepper to taste (the soy sauce should give enough salt). For bites, roll teaspoonfuls into balls. For burgers, take tablespoonfuls and squish into a patty shape. You can use a cookie cutter on the patties to create star-shaped burgers. If you have time, put them on a plate and chill for 1 hour or preferably overnight. However, they can be coated and cooked without chilling.

Mix together the dried bread crumbs and the remaining 2 tablespoons Parmesan on a large plate, along with salt and pepper to taste. Put the flour on a plate and season with salt and pepper. Beat the egg in a small bowl.

Dust the bites/burgers in the seasoned flour, then dip in the egg and roll in the bread crumbs. Heat the canola oil in a large nonstick frying pan and cook the bites/burgers for 1 to 2 minutes on each side, until golden. Drain on paper towels and serve warm—with buns, lettuce, tomato, and mayonnaise for burgers.

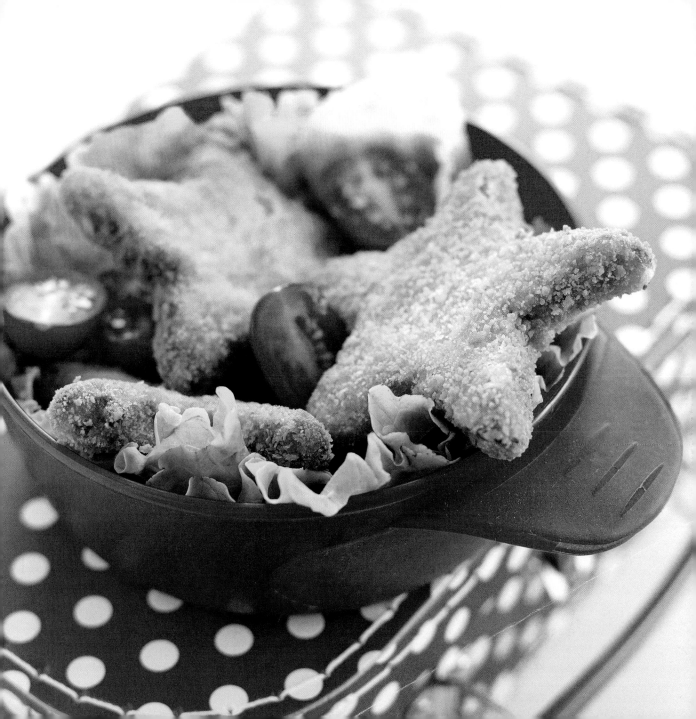

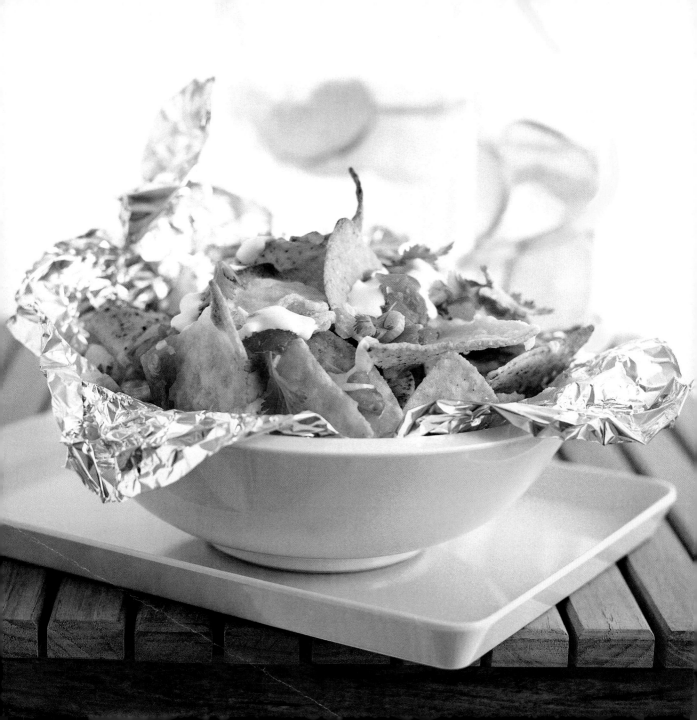

Nachos

I find that I have to make little individual portions of nachos, as my children always end up arguing over who is eating the most and this is the only way I can guarantee they all get the same! However, you can just pile the tortilla chips together in the center of the foil and sprinkle with the salsa and cheese, then broil and let the children help themselves. It is also really easy to make double quantities (or more) if you need to please a crowd. I like to make my own fresh salsa, but you can always use a quarter cup of your favorite store-bought one instead.

To make the salsa, mix all of the ingredients together in a small bowl, seasoning to taste with the salt and pepper. Cover and chill until needed—it will keep for up to 2 days in the fridge.

To make the nachos, preheat the broiler and line a broiler pan with foil. Spread the tortilla chips on the foil and top each one with half a teaspoon of salsa and a little of the cheese. Broil for 1 to 2 minutes, until the cheese has just melted. Watch carefully, as the edges of the tortilla chips can burn easily.

Transfer the nachos to two plates and top each with a small blob of sour cream, if using. Serve immediately, with more salsa.

🍲 Preparation 10 minutes
🕐 Cook 2 minutes
🍥 Makes 2 portions
❄ Not suitable for freezing or reheating

For the mild salsa
1 large tomato, peeled, seeded, and diced
1 scallion, thinly sliced
2 teaspoons chopped fresh cilantro (or to taste)
1 teaspoon fresh lime juice
salt and pepper, to season

For the nachos
12 plain tortilla chips
¹/₄ cup grated Cheddar
1 tablespoon sour cream (optional)

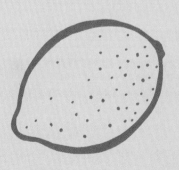
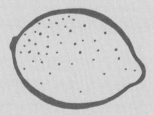

Tortilla Pizza Margherita

🍲 Preparation 5 minutes
🕐 Cook 9 minutes
🅖 Makes 1 portion
❄️ Not suitable for freezing
or reheating

one 7-inch flour tortilla
2 generous tablespoons tomato
  sauce
¹/₃ cup grated Cheddar or
  mozzarella

**Toppings Menu (I would suggest
no more than 2 toppings per
pizza, if using)**
2 or 3 pitted black olives, cut
  into rings
1 cherry or grape tomato, cut
  into rings
fresh basil leaves
2 cubes drained canned
  pineapple, cut into small dice
1 tablespoon diced red bell pepper
1 tablespoon drained canned
  corn
1 scallion, sliced
2 mushrooms, sliced and
  sautéed in a little oil
3 or 4 very thin slices zucchini,
  brushed with a little oil before
  putting on pizza
1 tablespoon freshly grated
  Parmesan
1 oil-packed sun-dried tomato,
  drained and finely chopped

I love thin-crust pizzas, and flour tortillas make an ideal "instant" base—turning deliciously crisp in the oven. They are also perfect for smaller children, who find the slimmer base easier to eat. Sometimes the air bubbles in the tortilla puff up a bit as the pizza bakes—but they deflate as soon as it comes out of the oven, so don't panic! You can use your favorite tomato sauce recipe or store-bought sauce, or try my recipe for Quick Tomato Sauce (page 32).

Preheat the oven to 400°F.

Put the tortilla on a baking sheet and spread with the tomato sauce. Sprinkle with the cheese. You can also add any toppings that your child may like (see suggestions, left). Bake for 8 to 9 minutes, until the cheese has melted and the base is crisp. Cut into triangles and allow to cool slightly before serving.

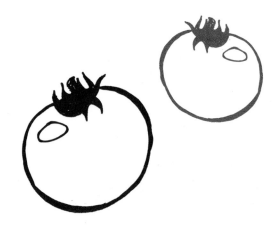

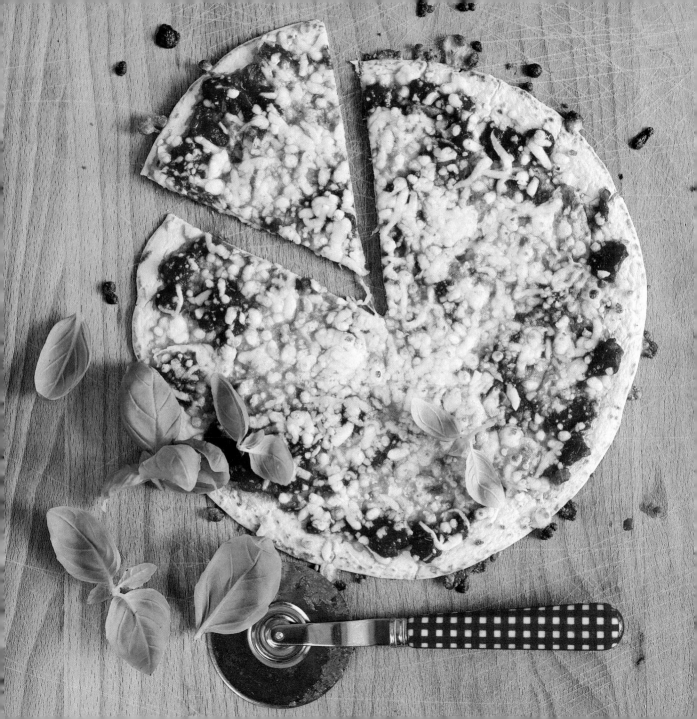

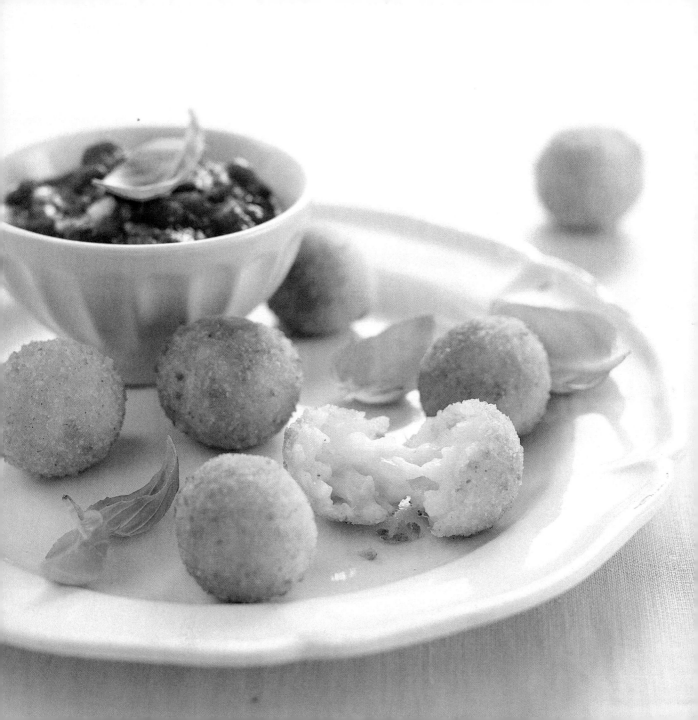

Arancini with Quick Tomato Sauce

Arancini are a popular snack in Italy and were originally invented by thrifty Italians to use up leftover risotto. I have used grated ordinary mozzarella here, as it is a bit drier than fresh mozzarella and helps to make the base mixture stickier.

Melt the butter in a large saucepan and sauté the shallot for 2 to 3 minutes, until translucent. Add the garlic and rice, and cook, stirring constantly, for 2 minutes more. Add 1²/₃ cups of the broth and bring to a boil, then reduce the heat to a simmer. Cook the rice for 20 to 25 minutes, until just tender. Stir every 4 to 5 minutes and add a little of the remaining broth if it becomes too dry.

Remove the pan from the heat and stir in the cheeses. Season to taste with a little pepper (you are unlikely to need extra salt). Spread the risotto out on a large plate and let cool, then cover and chill as quickly as possible.

Roll heaping teaspoonfuls of the cold risotto into balls. Season the bread crumbs with salt and pepper and a little paprika, if using. Put the flour on a plate and the egg in a small bowl. Dust the risotto balls with flour, dip in egg, and coat in bread crumbs, then put on a baking sheet lined with plastic wrap.

Put enough oil into a large frying pan to give a depth of ½ inch and put over medium heat. When the oil is shimmering, add the arancini and fry for 6 to 8 minutes, turning frequently, until golden brown. Drain on a plate lined with paper towels. Serve with tomato sauce (pages 32 and 33) for dipping.

☕ Preparation 15 minutes, plus cooling and chilling
🕐 Cook 25 minutes for rice, plus 16 minutes frying
🍽 Makes about 28 arancini, 7 to 9 portions (recipe is easily halved)
❄ Suitable for freezing: Cover the baking sheet with plastic wrap and freeze the arancini until firm, then transfer to a freezer bag. Cook directly from frozen on medium-low heat, increasing the cooking time to 10 to 12 minutes. Check that the centers are piping hot, then allow to cool slightly before serving.

1 tablespoon butter
1 small shallot, finely chopped
½ small garlic clove, crushed
heaping ½ cup risotto rice
scant 2¼ cups hot vegetable or chicken broth
⅓ cup grated mozzarella
⅓ cup grated sharp Cheddar
3 tablespoons freshly grated Parmesan
salt and pepper, to season
⅓ cup unseasoned dried bread crumbs
a pinch of paprika (optional)
2 tablespoons flour
1 egg, beaten
canola oil, for frying

Quick Tomato Sauce

🍲 Preparation 5 minutes
🕐 Cook 22 minutes
🍴 Makes 3 or 4 portions
❄ Suitable for freezing: Freeze in a resealable container. Thaw overnight in the fridge or for 1 to 2 hours at room temperature.

1 tablespoon olive oil
1 shallot, diced
1 garlic clove, crushed
one 14-ounce can diced tomatoes
1 teaspoon light brown sugar
1 tablespoon ketchup
salt and pepper, to season

Use half to accompany the arancini on page 31—the rest freezes well and can be served with pasta or used as a topping for pizza.

Heat the oil in a large frying pan, and sauté the shallot and garlic for 2 minutes, stirring constantly. Add the remaining ingredients and bring to a boil, squashing the tomatoes with the back of a wooden spoon. Boil, stirring frequently, for 15 minutes, or until the sauce has thickened.

Garlic and Herb Dip

🍲 Preparation 5 minutes
🍴 Makes 3 or 4 portions
❄ Not suitable for freezing or reheating

3 tablespoons mayonnaise
1 tablespoon Greek-style yogurt
1 teaspoon milk
1/4 teaspoon crushed garlic
1/4 teaspoon fresh lemon juice
1 teaspoon finely chopped fresh
   parsley (or you could use
   fresh cilantro or dill)
salt, for seasoning

Children tend to like garlic more than we might expect, and this dip is delicious with lots of things—bread sticks, carrot and cucumber sticks, Buffalo Wings (page 95), fish sticks or chicken nuggets (pages 58 and 77), and pita bread sticks.

Simply mix all the ingredients together with a pinch of salt. The dip will keep in the fridge for up to 3 days.

Grape Tomato Sauce

This would make a good dipping sauce for vegetarian dishes, such as Mini Vegetable Balls (page 53), Grilled Vegetable Skewers (page 36), Arancini (page 31), Veggie Bites/Burgers (page 24), and Baked Mozzarella Sticks (page 45), or for non-vegetarians, the Krispie Chicken Nuggets (page 77) and Annabel's Chicken Croquettes (page 80).

Preheat the oven to 350°F.

Halve the grape tomatoes and put in a small baking dish. Sprinkle with the thyme leaves and drizzle with 1 tablespoon of the olive oil. Tuck the garlic in the center and roast for 20 minutes.

Meanwhile, sauté the shallot in the remaining 1 tablespoon oil for 5 minutes. Add the canned tomatoes, tomato paste, ketchup, and sugar, and simmer for 10 minutes. Add the roasted tomatoes and garlic and cook for 30 minutes more. Whiz in a food processor or blender. If you want a very smooth sauce, press this through a strainer.

⊙ Preparation 10 minutes
🕐 Cook 50 minutes
🍴 Makes 4 portions
❄ Suitable for freezing and reheating. Let cool and freeze in a resealable container. Thaw at room temperature for 2 to 3 hours or in a microwave for 2 to 3 minutes. Can be reheated over gentle heat for 5 minutes, or for approximately 2 minutes in a microwave.

one 1-pint container grape
   tomatoes
1/4 teaspoon fresh thyme leaves
2 tablespoons olive oil
1 garlic clove, halved
1 large shallot, diced
one 14-ounce can diced
   tomatoes
2 tablespoons tomato paste
1 tablespoon ketchup
1 teaspoon sugar

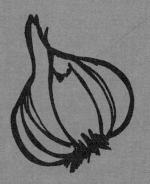
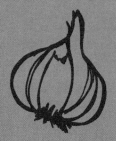

Potato Pizzette Bites

🍽 Preparation 5 minutes
🕐 Cook 25 minutes
🍴 Makes 2 portions (easily doubled)
❄️ Not suitable for freezing or reheating

1 large waxy-type potato (Yukon gold, or similar), skin on and washed thoroughly
1 tablespoon olive oil
salt and pepper, to season
3 tablespoons tomato sauce, such as Quick Tomato Sauce (page 32)
½ cup grated Cheddar or mozzarella

Slices of crisp potato make an unusual base for small pizzas or pizzette. Sautéed red onion and fresh thyme are additional tasty toppings.

Preheat the oven to 400°F.

Cut 8 large slices of potato, each around 1/12 inch thick, cutting crosswise from the center of the potato. You won't need the thinner end bits of the potato, but these will keep for up to 2 days in the fridge, covered with cold water, and can be used for mashed or boiled potatoes.

Brush each potato slice with the oil and season with a little salt and pepper. Lay the slices on a baking sheet lined with parchment paper and bake for 10 minutes. Turn the slices over and bake for 8 to 10 minutes more, until golden and crisp. Watch carefully for the last 2 to 3 minutes.

Top each potato slice with around 1 teaspoon of the tomato sauce and sprinkle with the cheese. Bake for 5 to 7 minutes more or broil for 2 to 3 minutes, until the cheese has melted. Let cool slightly before serving.

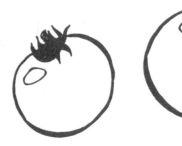

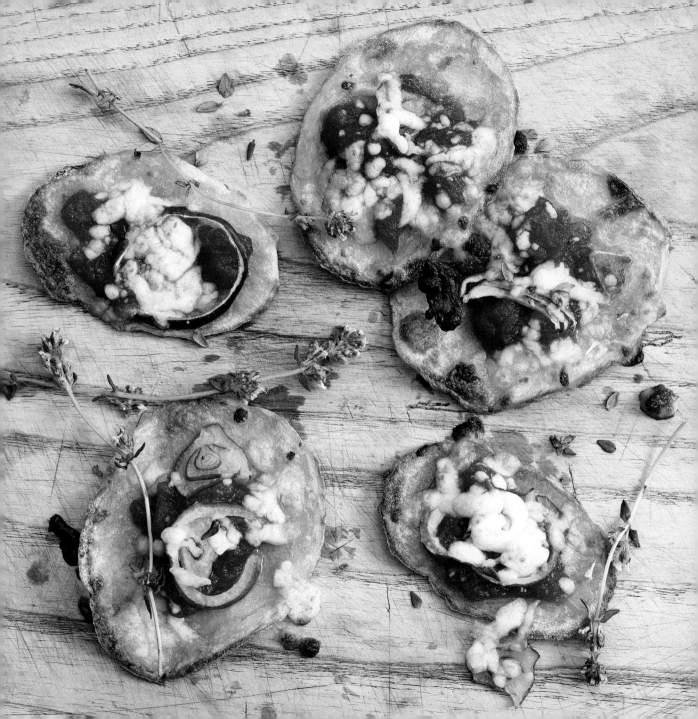

Grilled Vegetable Skewers

🍲 Preparation 8 minutes,
plus marinating
🕐 Cook 10 minutes
🍲 Makes 4 skewers, 2 to 4
portions
☺ Suitable for children under 1
❄ Not suitable for freezing or
reheating but can be eaten cold

1 large red bell pepper
1 large yellow or orange bell
    pepper
½ medium green zucchini
½ medium yellow squash (or
    more zucchini if unavailable)

For the marinade
2 tablespoons olive oil
2 teaspoons balsamic vinegar
1 teaspoon sugar
salt and pepper, to season

You will also need 4 wooden
    skewers, soaked in warm
    water for 30 minutes

Marinating the vegetables in a balsamic vinaigrette helps to accentuate their natural sweetness and can make them more appealing to kids. The vegetables are delicious warm, and leftovers are yummy added to tomato pasta sauces or to salads (see my Mix 'n' Match Pasta Salad, page 117).

Cut off the tops of the bell peppers and remove the cores and seeds. Cut into rings. Slice 4 circles from each squash, approximately ¼ inch thick, and cut each circle across in half to give 8 semicircles each of green and yellow squash.

Put the marinade ingredients into a medium bowl and whisk together, seasoning to taste with the salt and pepper. Add the vegetables and toss to coat. Marinate for a minimum of 2 hours, or overnight, stirring the vegetables occasionally.

Preheat the broiler and line a broiler pan with foil. Thread pieces of bell pepper and squash onto the skewers. Put the skewers on the foil and brush with some of the remaining marinade. Broil for 4 to 5 minutes, until the vegetables start to soften around the edges—watch carefully, as they can brown very quickly if they are too close to the heat source.

Turn the skewers over and brush with more marinade. Broil for 4 to 5 minutes more, until the vegetables are cooked through. Again watch carefully; you want the vegetables to brown without burning. The skewers can also be grilled over medium-hot coals.

Allow the skewers to cool slightly before serving. Leftover vegetables can be removed from the skewers and stored, covered, in the fridge for up to 2 days.

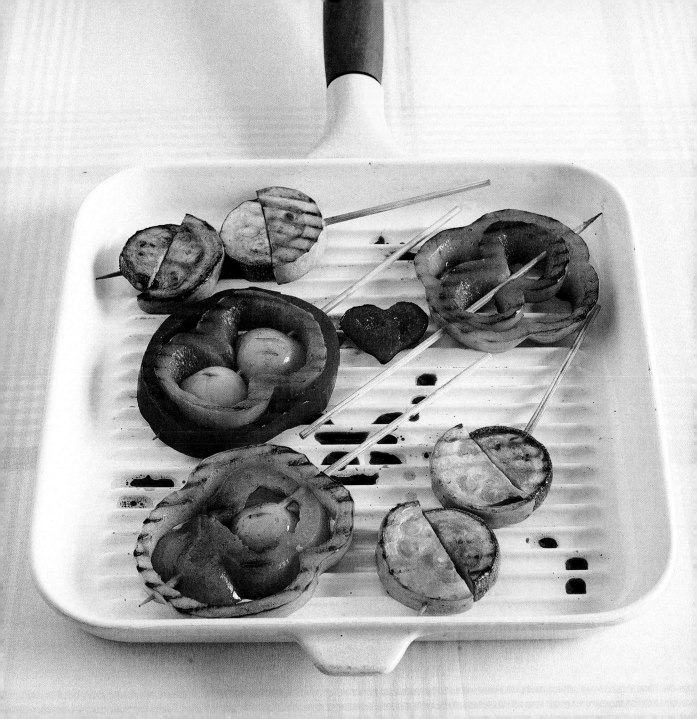

Petit Panini

🍲 Preparation 5 minutes
🕐 Cook 7 minutes
🥄 Makes 1 portion (for an older child)
❄️ Not suitable for freezing or reheating

1 tablespoon butter, softened
1 hot dog roll, split through the side
2 slices tomato
2 slices mozzarella
salt and pepper, to season
1 teaspoon olive oil

Panini are delicious Italian toasted sandwiches, usually made with small loaves of bread. I like to use hot dog rolls, as they are a perfect size for children.

Spread the butter on the cut sides of the roll. Lay the tomato and mozzarella on the base of the roll, season, and make into a sandwich using the top of the roll. Preheat a grill pan and grease with the olive oil. Put the panini, top side down, on the grill pan and press down well with a spatula. Cook for 3 to 4 minutes, until golden and crisp. Turn over the panini and cook for 3 minutes more, until warmed through. Cut in half and serve.

Falafel with Minty Yogurt Dressing

🍲 Preparation 20 minutes
🕐 Cook 8 minutes (assuming 2 batches)
🥄 Makes 4 to 6 portions
❄️ Not suitable for freezing but can be reheated in a microwave for approximately 1 minute; also good cold

1 small onion, finely chopped
1 tablespoon olive oil
1 small garlic clove, crushed
¼ to ½ teaspoon ground cumin

As with meat eaters, the key to a healthy vegetarian diet is to eat a wide range of foods. This is particularly true for vegetarians, because apart from a few foods like quinoa and tofu, most plant proteins are not complete, and only by eating a variety of them can you optimize your protein intake. Falafel is equally delicious cold, so it is a good lunch box option. Garbanzo beans (also called chickpeas) are a good source of vegetable protein.

Sauté the onion in the olive oil for 8 to 10 minutes, until soft. Add the garlic, cumin, and coriander, and cook for 2 minutes more. While the onion is cooking, drain the garbanzo beans and rinse with cold water. Turn the garbanzo beans onto paper towels and rub dry, then transfer to a bowl, leaving behind as many of the papery skins as possible.

Mash the garbanzo beans with a potato masher, then stir in the sautéed onion, the parsley, lemon zest, and hummus, and season to taste with salt and pepper. Divide the mixture into 12 scant tablespoons, roll firmly into balls, then press slightly to make small burger shapes. Dust with the flour and pat off any excess.

Heat the canola oil in a large frying pan and fry the falafel for 1 to 1½ minutes on each side, until golden. Drain briefly on paper towels.

To make the dressing, mix together the yogurt, mint, and lemon juice with the salt. (The dressing and cooked falafel can be stored, covered, in the fridge for 2 days.)

Toast and split the pitas or warm the wraps or tortillas. Spread with a tablespoon of the yogurt dressing, and add 2 falafels and a little lettuce, if using. You can serve these with extra lemon wedges to squeeze over.

¼ to ½ teaspoon ground coriander
one 15-ounce can garbanzo beans (chickpeas)
1½ teaspoons chopped fresh parsley
finely grated zest of 1 small lemon
3 tablespoons hummus
salt and pepper, to season
1 tablespoon flour
3 tablespoons canola oil, for frying

For the minty yogurt dressing
⅓ cup Greek-style yogurt
1 teaspoon chopped fresh mint (10 to 12 leaves)
1 teaspoon fresh lemon juice
a pinch of salt

4 to 6 pita breads, flatbread wraps, or 7-inch flour tortillas, shredded lettuce, and lemon wedges, to serve (optional)

TIP
You can change it up a bit by using different varieties of hummus (e.g., roasted red bell pepper). I have suggested serving these in a wrap or pita if warm, but you can also just serve them on their own, in which case you need to add a tablespoon of milk to the yogurt to make the dressing a little thinner.

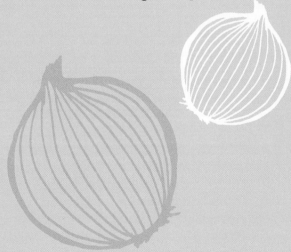

Mushroom Pâté

🍲 Preparation 8 minutes,
plus cooling
🕐 Cook 12 minutes
🍴 Makes 4 portions
❄ Not suitable for freezing
or reheating

1 tablespoon olive oil
8 ounces mushrooms,
   thinly sliced
1 small garlic clove, crushed
¼ teaspoon fresh lemon juice
2 ounces cream cheese or
   Neufchâtel cheese
salt and pepper, to season

Children who won't normally eat mushrooms may try this pâté if they don't know what is in it! It is also a great option for vegetarians. I like it best spread thinly on fresh hot toast.

Heat the oil in a large frying pan and sauté the mushrooms for 8 to 10 minutes, until they are soft and any liquid released has evaporated. Add the garlic and cook for 2 minutes more. Transfer the mushrooms to a food processor and allow to cool to room temperature.

Whiz the cooled mushrooms until finely chopped, then add the lemon juice and cheese and whiz again to form a smooth pâté. Season to taste with salt and pepper, then transfer to a container, cover, and chill until needed. The pâté will keep for up to 3 days in the fridge.

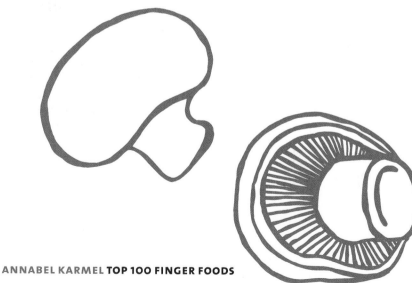

Oven-Baked Potato Wedges

Oven-baked potato wedges are a healthy alternative to french fries—I have left the skin on the potato, as it contains a lot of extra vitamins and fiber. You can make spicy wedges by adding the optional paprika or fajita seasoning. These are particularly good served with my Garlic and Herb Dip (page 32).

Preheat the oven to 400°F.

Cut the potato lengthwise into 8 wedges. Put the oil in a bowl and season with a little salt and pepper plus the paprika or fajita seasoning, if using (for spicy wedges). Add the wedges and toss them in the oil.

Lay the wedges on a baking sheet lined with parchment paper and bake for 10 minutes. Turn them over and bake for 10 minutes more. Turn over again and bake for another 5 to 10 minutes, until the wedges are golden and cooked through.

Let cool slightly before serving. Can be stored in the fridge, cooked, for 1 day. Reheat for 5 minutes in an oven preheated to 400°F.

🍲 Preparation 5 minutes
🕐 Cook 30 minutes
🌐 Makes 2 portions (easily doubled)
❄ Not suitable for freezing but can be reheated for 5 minutes in an oven preheated to 400°F

1 medium potato, such as Yukon gold, skin on and washed thoroughly
1½ teaspoons olive oil
salt and pepper, to season
¼ teaspoon paprika or fajita seasoning (optional)

TIP
I line the baking sheet with parchment paper, as otherwise the wedges tend to stick to the sheet. I have left the spicing as optional, as not everyone will like it. You may prefer to prepare half the wedges spiced and half plain.

Cheese and Tomato Mini Quiches

🍲 Preparation 20 minutes
🕐 Cook 20 minutes
🍥 Makes 8 mini quiches
❄ Suitable for freezing: Freeze baked and chilled quiches in a resealable container. Thaw overnight in the fridge. Reheat for 20 to 30 seconds in a microwave or for 8 to 10 minutes in an oven preheated to 300°F.

one 7½-ounce store-bought refrigerated piecrust
8 cherry or grape tomatoes
1 egg
⅓ cup milk
1 tablespoon cream or extra milk
2 tablespoons freshly grated Parmesan
salt and pepper, to season
scant ½ cup grated sharp Cheddar

I like to use cherry or grape tomatoes in these little quiches, as they are deliciously sweet and complement the cheesy filling well. For smaller children, you can serve the quiches cut into quarters.

Preheat the oven to 400°F.

Use a 3½-inch round cookie cutter to cut out 8 pastry circles (reroll trimmings if necessary) from the piecrust. Press the pastry carefully into eight cups of a regular muffin pan and chill for 10 minutes. Alternatively, you can make these in mini quiche pans.

Cut each cherry tomato into quarters and set aside. Beat together the egg, milk, cream, and Parmesan, and season with a little salt (the Parmesan is quite salty) and pepper. Put 4 tomato quarters in the base of each crust. Spoon in the egg mixture (approximately 1 tablespoon per quiche), then top with the Cheddar.

Bake for 20 minutes, or until the pastry is golden and the filling is set. Let cool in the pan for 10 minutes, then run a knife around the edge of each quiche and gently ease it out of the pan. Serve warm or cold. Can be kept in the fridge for up to 2 days.

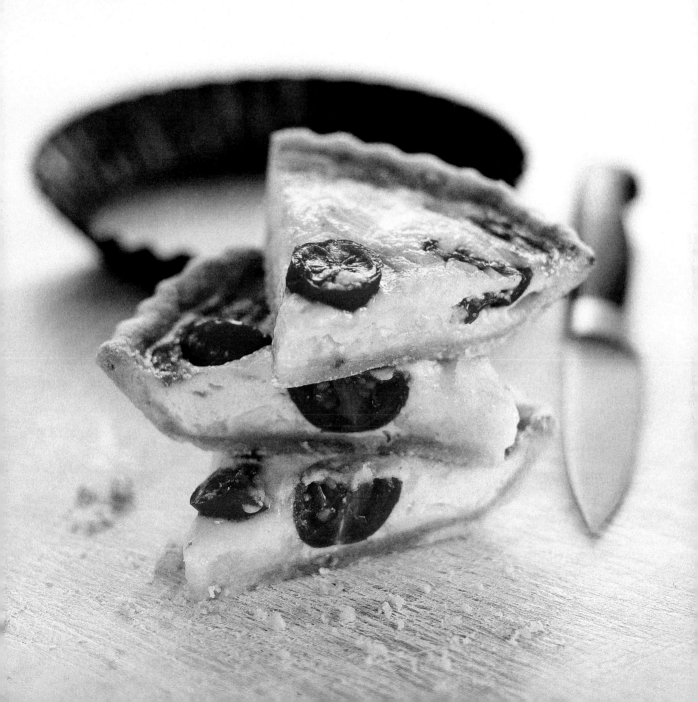

Sweet Corn Pancakes

🍲 Preparation 5 minutes
🕐 Cook 12 minutes (assuming 3 batches)
🥞 Makes 10 to 12 pancakes
❄️ Suitable for freezing and reheating: Put individual portions of 2 or 3 pancakes in a single layer on pieces of foil and fold up to make a packet. Freeze. To reheat from frozen, warm for 5 minutes in an oven preheated to 400°F.

1 cup drained canned corn
2 large scallions, quartered
1 egg
1 tablespoon honey
½ cup self-rising flour
a pinch of salt (optional)
2 to 3 tablespoons canola oil, for frying

Whizzing the corn so that the pancakes aren't lumpy makes them much better for smaller children. It also results in a slightly thicker batter, which makes the pancakes more robust and so more suitable as finger food. They are delicious for breakfast or lunch, or as a snack.

Put the corn and scallions in a food processor and whiz until finely chopped. Add the egg and honey, whiz again, add the flour and salt, if using, and pulse until combined. Transfer the batter to a pitcher.

Heat a little of the oil in a large nonstick frying pan. Drop tablespoonfuls of the batter into the pan and cook for 1½ to 2 minutes, until the underside is golden and bubbles are appearing on the surface of the pancakes. Flip the pancakes over using a spatula and cook for 1 to 2 minutes more, until golden. Let cool slightly before serving. You can also make tiny pancakes by cooking teaspoonfuls of batter. Pancakes can be kept in the fridge, cooked, for 2 days. Reheat for 10 to 15 seconds in a microwave or in a frying pan over gentle heat.

Baked Mozzarella Sticks

The key to making mozzarella sticks is to ensure a good coating of bread crumbs, which will prevent the cheese from melting all over the baking sheet. If you see any bald patches after crumb coating, dip that spot back in the egg and press on some extra bread crumbs. You can fry the sticks if you prefer: Omit the olive oil from the recipe and shallow-fry in oil over medium heat for 2 to 3 minutes per side.

Preheat the oven to 400°F.

Cut the mozzarella into 4 slices; the slices should be about 1/2 inch thick. Cut each slice lengthwise into quarters to get 16 sticks. (If using balls of fresh mozzarella, pat off any excess water with paper towels.)

Put the bread crumbs in a bowl and mix in the Parmesan, paprika, and salt and pepper to taste, then stir in the oil, using a fork and making sure the oil is distributed evenly. Beat the eggs in a medium bowl.

Dip 2 or 3 mozzarella sticks into the egg and carefully roll in the bread crumbs. Dip in the egg again and roll in a second coat of bread crumbs, making sure the mozzarella is well covered. Put the coated sticks on a baking sheet lined with parchment paper. Repeat with the remaining mozzarella.

Bake the sticks for 4 minutes, turn, and bake for 3 to 4 minutes more, until the bread crumbs are turning golden. Don't worry if a little mozzarella melts out. Remove from the oven and let the sticks stand for 5 to 6 minutes, to allow the cheese to cool and firm up slightly. Meanwhile, warm the tomato sauce.

Serve the sticks with cups of the tomato sauce for dunking. For smaller children, it may help to cut each stick into 2 or 3 pieces.

Preparation 15 minutes
Cook 8 minutes
Makes 16 sticks, about 3 portions
Suitable for freezing: Put the sticks on a baking sheet lined with plastic wrap. Cover with more plastic wrap and freeze for 3 to 4 hours, until firm. Transfer to freezer bags and use within 1 month. Bake directly from frozen, increasing the baking time to 10 to 11 minutes and turning halfway through. Suitable for reheating; heat in the oven for about 6 minutes or until hot.

5 ounces firm mozzarella
1 cup unseasoned dried bread
   crumbs
1/3 cup freshly grated Parmesan
1 teaspoon paprika
salt and pepper, to season
4 teaspoons olive oil
2 eggs
1/2 cup tomato sauce, to serve
   (try Quick Tomato Sauce,
   page 32, or use your favorite)

Baked Parsnip and Sweet Potato Chips

🍲 Preparation 8 minutes
🕐 Cook 15 to 20 minutes
🍥 Makes 4 portions
❄ Not suitable for freezing
or reheating

1 small parsnip, peeled
1 tablespoon olive oil
½ small sweet potato, peeled
a pinch of salt (optional)

TIP
The parsnip and potato cook at slightly different rates, so it is easier to cook them on separate baking sheets. Watch them carefully toward the end of the cooking time.

Kids who don't always like vegetables may be fooled into eating these chips, as they are naturally slightly sweet and very delicious. And they are healthier, too, as they are baked rather than fried. They would be a nice accompaniment for Veggie Bites/Burgers (page 24).

Preheat the oven to 300°F. Line two large baking sheets with parchment paper.

Use a small swivel peeler to peel thin strips from the parsnip. Put the strips in a bowl and toss with 1½ teaspoons of the oil. Spread out in a single layer on one of the prepared baking sheets. Do the same with the sweet potato, spreading the strips on the second baking sheet.

Bake for 10 minutes, then rotate the baking sheets. Bake for 5 minutes more, then check and remove from the oven if crisp and browned at the edges. Otherwise, continue cooking for 4 to 5 minutes more, checking every minute, as the chips can go brown very quickly. You may find that the parsnip cooks slightly more quickly than the potato.

Transfer the cooked chips to a bowl and sprinkle with salt, if you like. These are best served the day they are made but can be stored in an airtight container overnight (they may soften a bit).

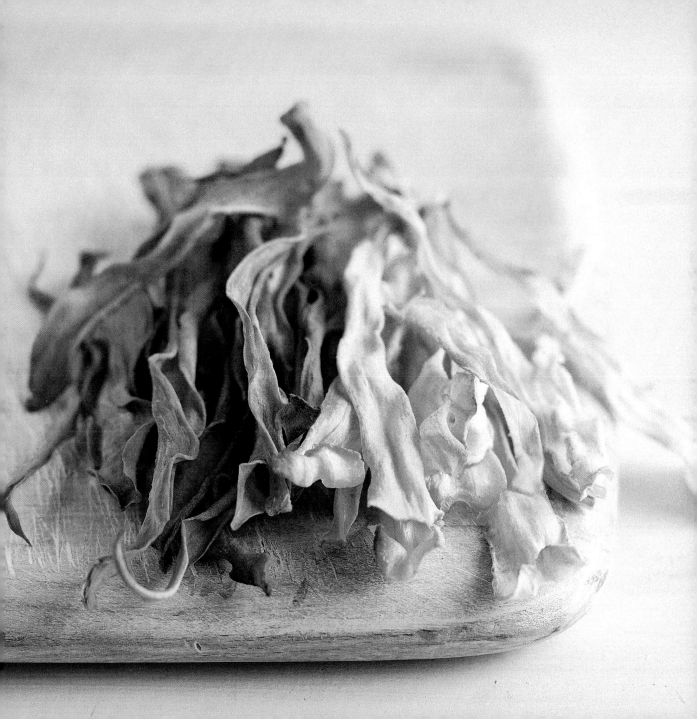

Cottage Cheese Dip

Preparation 5 minutes
Makes 5 or 6 portions
Not suitable for freezing

1 cup cottage cheese
¼ cup mayonnaise
2 heaping tablespoons ketchup
¼ teaspoon fresh lemon juice
a tiny drop of Worcestershire
    sauce (optional)

Cottage cheese is a great source of calcium, but many children don't like the texture. However, whizzing the cheese until smooth can make it the base for a yummy dip.

Put all the ingredients in a food processor and whiz until smooth. Transfer to a bowl, cover, and store in the fridge until ready to use. This would make a good dipping sauce for sticks of cucumber, carrot, and red bell pepper. If you want to prepare the vegetables in advance, wrap them in damp paper towels and store in the fridge to keep them fresh.

Variation: Cottage Cheese with Swirled Fruit Puree

Blend the cottage cheese with a little sugar and vanilla extract, and swirl in some store-bought apricot puree or preserves such as Bonne Maman.

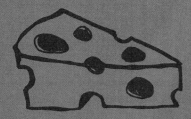

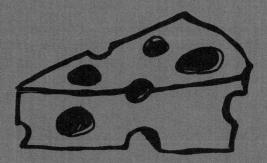

Baked Baby Potatoes

Stuffed baked potatoes are usually popular with older children but are a bit unwieldy for little ones. Small new potatoes (or use fingerlings or small blue-, purple-, or red-fleshed potatoes) make a perfect alternative for a finger-sized version!

Preheat the oven to 400°F.

Put the potatoes into a medium bowl, drizzle with the oil, and season with a little salt and pepper. Toss to coat the potatoes with the oil, then transfer to a baking sheet. Bake for 30 to 35 minutes, until the potatoes are cooked through.

Remove the potatoes from the oven and let cool slightly, then cut in half and carefully scoop out some of the center with a teaspoon. Put the scooped potato flesh into a small bowl and add the sour cream and chives. Mash together thoroughly and season to taste with salt and pepper.

Spoon the filling into the potato skins and sprinkle with the cheese, if using. Return to the baking sheet and bake for 5 to 10 minutes, until heated through.

Suitable for reheating: The filled potatoes can be chilled overnight, then reheated in a 400°F oven for 15 to 20 minutes, but they do not reheat well after they have been stuffed and baked, as they can be a little dry.

🍳 Preparation 10 minutes
🕐 Cook 45 minutes
🥘 Makes 4 portions (older children)
❄ Not suitable for freezing, but suitable for reheating

8 small new potatoes, such as creamer, Yukon gold, or Red Bliss, scrubbed
1 teaspoon olive oil
salt and pepper, to season
3 tablespoons sour cream or crème fraîche
1 teaspoon snipped fresh chives, or 1 small scallion, finely chopped
⅓ cup grated cheese (optional)

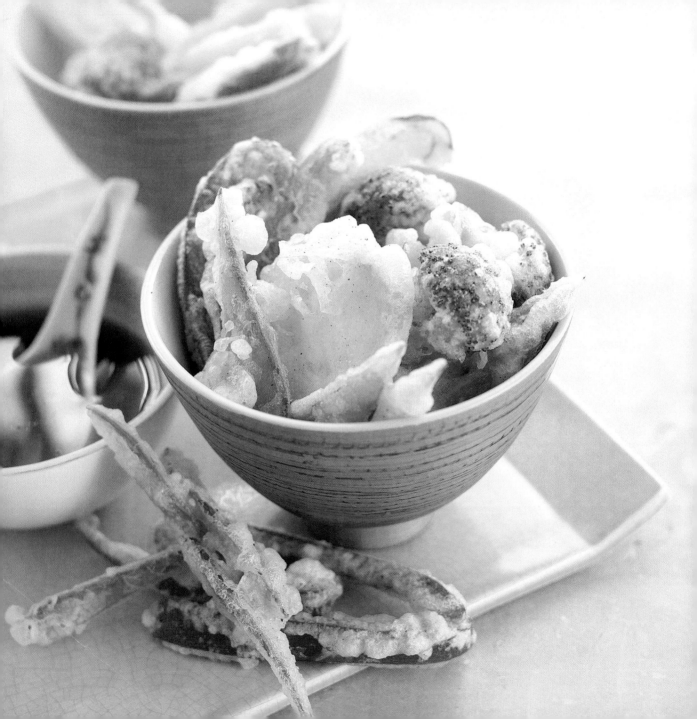

Vegetable Tempura

Crisp tempura batter is usually a good way to tempt sworn veggie haters to take a taste. To keep the batter light, mix it as quickly as possible and don't worry if there are a few lumps.

Stir the dipping sauce ingredients together until the sugar has dissolved. Divide among four small dipping bowls and set aside.

Have all of the vegetables prepared before you make the batter. You can prepare them a couple of hours in advance and keep them on a plate in the fridge, covered with a damp paper towel and then wrapped with plastic wrap.

Put the oil in a large, deep saucepan (it should not come more than halfway up the sides of the pan) or deep-fat fryer. Heat the oil to 375°F. Line a couple of baking sheets with a double layer of paper towels.

Put the flour and cornstarch in a large bowl and whisk together with a fork. Add the sparkling water and mix quickly with the fork—don't worry if there are a few lumps. The batter should be the consistency of half-and-half; if it is too thick, add an extra 1 to 2 tablespoons of sparkling water.

Drop 5 or 6 pieces of the prepared vegetables into the batter, then gently put them one by one into the hot oil. Don't overcrowd the pan, or the oil will get too cold and the batter will be greasy. Fry for 2 to 3 minutes, turning once, until puffed and crisp and turning slightly golden at the edges. Use a slotted spoon to transfer the cooked vegetables to the baking sheets and let them drain for 1 to 2 minutes. Meanwhile, continue dipping and cooking the remainder of the vegetables. The tempura is best eaten within a few minutes of being cooked, but can be kept warm for 10 to 15 minutes in an oven preheated to 250°F.

Preparation 20 minutes
Cook 15 to 20 minutes
Makes 4 portions

For the dipping sauce
2 tablespoons mirin
1 tablespoon soy sauce (reduced sodium is fine)
1 tablespoon water
1/2 teaspoon sugar

1/2 red bell pepper, seeded and cut into thin strips
1 small yellow squash (or zucchini if unavailable), cut into 1/4-inch-thick rounds
1 small head broccoli, broken into bite-size florets
a handful of snow peas, trimmed
2 cups vegetable oil, for deep-frying
1 cup flour
1/2 cup cornstarch
1 cup sparkling water or soda water

TIP
You can also test the heat of the oil by dropping a cube of bread into the oil—if it is the correct temperature, the bread should turn golden brown in around 20 seconds.

Cheese and "Onion" Sandwich

🍲 Preparation 5 minutes
🕑 Makes 1 portion
❄ Not suitable for freezing

2 or 3 fresh chives, finely snipped
1 tablespoon mayonnaise
1 teaspoon water
scant ½ cup grated Cheddar
   (mild or sharp, according to
   your child's preference)
2 slices bread
1 tablespoon butter, softened

Onions can be a bit strong for smaller children, but the milder taste of chives makes a standard cheese sandwich a little more interesting. Rolling the bread makes a thin sandwich that smaller children find easier to eat.

Mix the chives, mayonnaise, and water together in a small bowl, then add the cheese and stir to combine.

Roll the slices of bread with a rolling pin until they are about half of their original thickness. Spread one side of each slice with a little of the butter. Spoon the cheese filling onto one of the buttered slices and sandwich with the second slice, pressing down well. Trim off the crusts and cut into squares or triangles to serve.

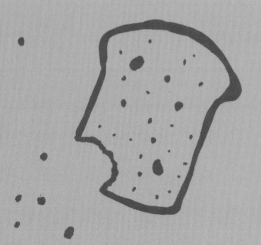

Mini Vegetable Balls

The combination of the sautéed red onion and grated carrot mixed with vegetables and flavored with Gruyère, Parmesan, and balsamic vinegar with a touch of soy sauce is bound to please everyone in the family. For older children, these would make delicious burgers and a nice change from beef burgers.

Heat the oil in a frying pan and sauté the vegetables for 8 minutes. Add the thyme and garlic and cook for 2 minutes. The vegetables should be fairly dry. Add the balsamic vinegar and cook for 30 seconds to 1 minute, until evaporated. Turn off the heat and stir in the sugar. Let cool slightly.

Put the bread in a food processor and whiz into crumbs. Add the vegetables, Gruyère, 2 tablespoons of the Parmesan, and the soy sauce, and season with pepper, then whiz until combined. Roll teaspoonfuls into balls. For bigger kids, form tablespoonfuls into burgers.

Mix the dried bread crumbs and remaining 3 tablespoons Parmesan on a plate with a little pepper. Put the flour on a separate plate and the egg in a bowl. Toss the balls in the flour, dip in the egg, and coat in the bread crumbs. (You may freeze them uncooked; put in a resealable container.)

Heat the canola oil in a frying pan and fry the balls for approximately 2 minutes, turning occasionally, or fry the burgers for about 2 minutes on each side. Drain on paper towels and let cool to warm before serving. (If frozen, cook from frozen; add 1 minute to the cooking time.)

Preparation 20 minutes
Cook 2 minutes (balls), 4 minutes (burgers)
Makes 27 balls
Suitable for children under 1
Suitable for freezing and reheating

1 tablespoon olive oil
1 small red onion, finely chopped
1 small carrot, peeled and finely grated
3 mushrooms, diced
½ small zucchini, grated
3 broccoli florets, chopped into small pieces
¼ teaspoon fresh thyme leaves
1 garlic clove, crushed
1 tablespoon balsamic vinegar
1 teaspoon light brown sugar
1 slice white bread, crusts removed
⅓ cup grated Gruyère
5 tablespoons freshly grated Parmesan
1½ teaspoons soy sauce
pepper, to season
3 tablespoons unseasoned dried bread crumbs
4½ teaspoons flour
1 egg, beaten with a pinch of salt (omit salt for those under 1)
3 to 4 tablespoons canola oil, for frying

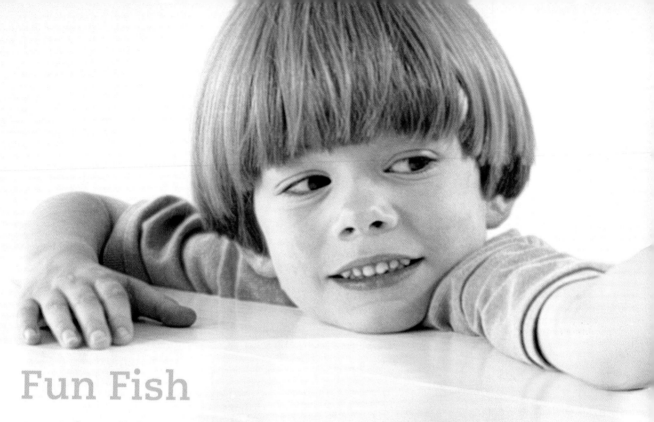

Fun Fish

Apart from fish being quick to cook and a fantastic source of protein, the omega-3s in oily fish are important for boosting brainpower. Making sure children get enough omega-3s can also revolutionize the lives of parents coping with youngsters who have dyslexia, ADHD (attention-deficit/hyperactivity disorder), and problems with motor skill development. There is overwhelming evidence that increasing omega-3 intake can result in improved concentration, learning, and behavior. Ideally, children should have two portions of oily fish a week (but not more, as there are concerns over levels of toxins).

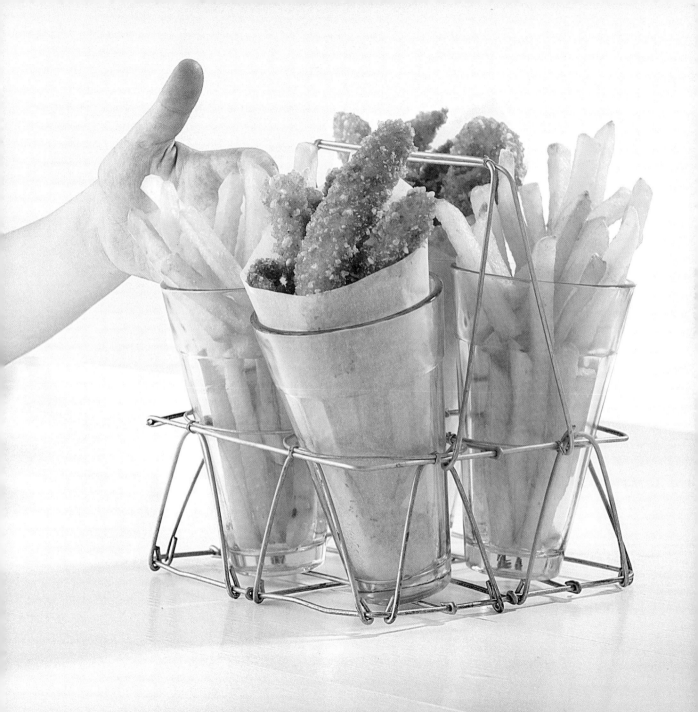

Salmon Fish Cakes

🍲 Preparation 10 minutes
🕐 Cook 5 minutes
🍥 Makes 12 fish cakes
☺ Suitable for children under 1
❄ Not recommended for freezing or reheating: Uncooked mixture can be stored, covered, in the fridge for 2 to 3 days.

one 7.5-ounce can red salmon, drained
2 slices white bread, crusts removed
2 scallions, finely chopped
2 tablespoons ketchup
1 teaspoon fresh lemon juice
1 tablespoon mayonnaise
salt and pepper, to season
2 to 3 tablespoons canola oil, for frying
2 tablespoons flour

Fish cakes are often an easy way to encourage toddlers to eat fish. You could also make these using cooked and flaked fresh salmon.

Remove the skin and any large bones from the salmon. Whiz the bread in a food processor to make into bread crumbs. Combine the flaked salmon, bread crumbs, scallions, ketchup, and lemon juice in a bowl. Add the mayonnaise a teaspoon at a time until the mixture binds together (you may not need it at all). Mix well and season with salt and pepper.

Heat the oil in a frying pan. Put the flour in a small bowl and season with salt and pepper. Roll tablespoonfuls of the mixture into balls. Roll the balls in the flour, flatten in the pan with the back of a spoon or a spatula, and fry for 4 to 5 minutes, turning occasionally. Drain on paper towels and let cool slightly before serving.

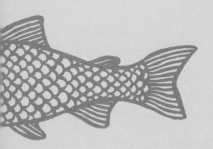

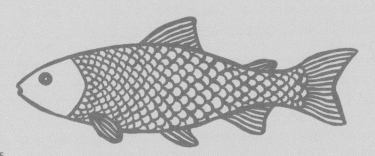

Marinated Shrimp with Tomato Salsa

Shrimp with a tasty dip make good finger food for the whole family, and the beauty of these is they are so quick to cook.

Put the shrimp in a small bowl and add the lime juice, cilantro, soy sauce, and pepper. Chill for a minimum of 30 minutes, but no longer than 1 hour, as the lime juice will start to "cook" the shrimp.

Meanwhile, make the salsa. Mix together all the ingredients except the cilantro and store in the fridge until needed.

Remove the shrimp from the marinade and pat dry. Heat the oil in a frying pan and fry the shrimp for about 90 seconds. Add 1 tablespoon of the marinade and allow to evaporate. Turn over the shrimp and fry for 90 seconds more, then add another tablespoon of the marinade and allow to evaporate. Check that the shrimp are cooked through by cutting into the fattest part of one.

When the shrimp are cooked, stir the chopped cilantro, if using, into the salsa and serve immediately.

Preparation 15 minutes, plus 30 minutes marinating
Cook 3 minutes
Makes 2 or 3 portions
Not suitable for freezing or reheating

5 ounces raw large shrimp, peeled and deveined
juice of 1 large lime
1 teaspoon roughly chopped fresh cilantro
1 teaspoon soy sauce
pepper, to season

For the tomato salsa
1 tablespoon finely chopped red onion
2 tomatoes, quartered, seeded, and finely diced
2 tablespoons olive oil
1 teaspoon soy sauce
1 teaspoon rice vinegar
1 teaspoon fresh lime juice
1 tablespoon chopped fresh cilantro (optional)

1 tablespoon canola oil, for frying

Krispie Fish "Fingers" with Lemon Mayo Dip

🍲 Preparation 20 minutes
🕐 Cook 4 minutes
🍽 Makes 6 to 8 portions
❄ Suitable for freezing: Lay the uncooked fish sticks on a baking sheet lined with plastic wrap. Cover with plastic wrap and freeze for 2 hours, or until firm. Transfer to freezer bags. Cook directly from frozen as described. Not suitable for reheating.

½ pound skinless flounder or sole fillets
1½ cups Rice Krispies
3 tablespoons freshly grated Parmesan
¼ teaspoon paprika
salt and pepper, to season
1 teaspoon sesame seeds (optional)
1 egg
2 tablespoons flour
2 to 3 tablespoons canola oil, for frying

For the dip
2 tablespoons mayonnaise
2 tablespoons Greek-style yogurt
1 teaspoon fresh lemon juice
a pinch of salt, to season (optional)

Rice Krispies make a tasty coating for fish, and I like to make these finger-size sticks, as they cook quickly and can be easily cooked from frozen. Another good coating to try is crushed cornflakes. Simply cut the fish into strips, coat in seasoned flour, lightly beaten egg, and crushed cornflakes, and sauté until golden and cooked through.

Cut the fish into pieces the size of a little finger. Cover and set aside in the fridge. Put the Rice Krispies, Parmesan, and paprika in a food processor and whiz to fine crumbs. Transfer to a plate, and stir in salt and pepper to taste and the sesame seeds, if using. Beat the egg in a bowl with a pinch of salt. Spread the flour on a separate plate.

Toss 3 or 4 of the fish pieces in the flour, dunk in the egg, and roll in the crumbs until well coated. Set aside on a clean plate and continue with the remaining fish. Cook immediately or freeze according to the instructions on the left.

Heat the oil in a large frying pan and add the fish sticks. Fry for 1½ to 2 minutes on each side, until golden and cooked through. Transfer to a plate lined with paper towels to cool slightly before serving.

To make the dip, mix all of the ingredients together in a small bowl. Serve with the fish sticks.

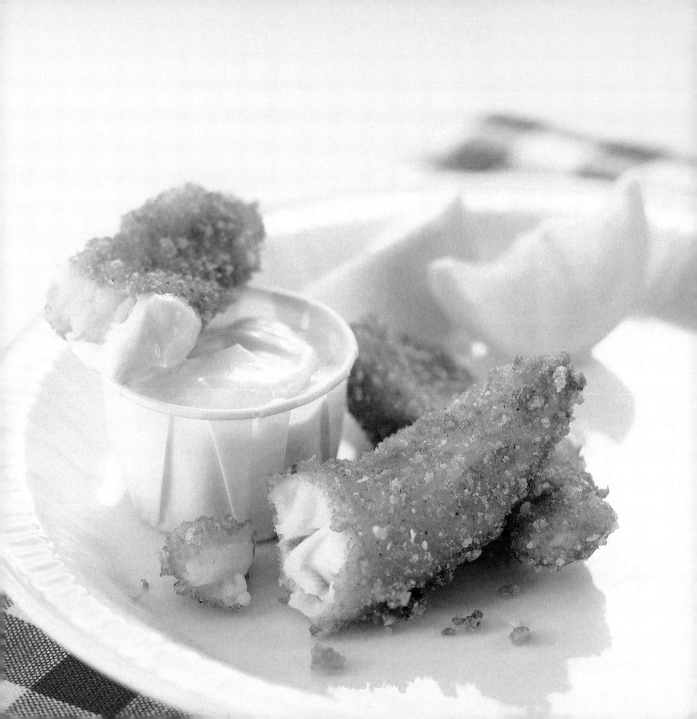

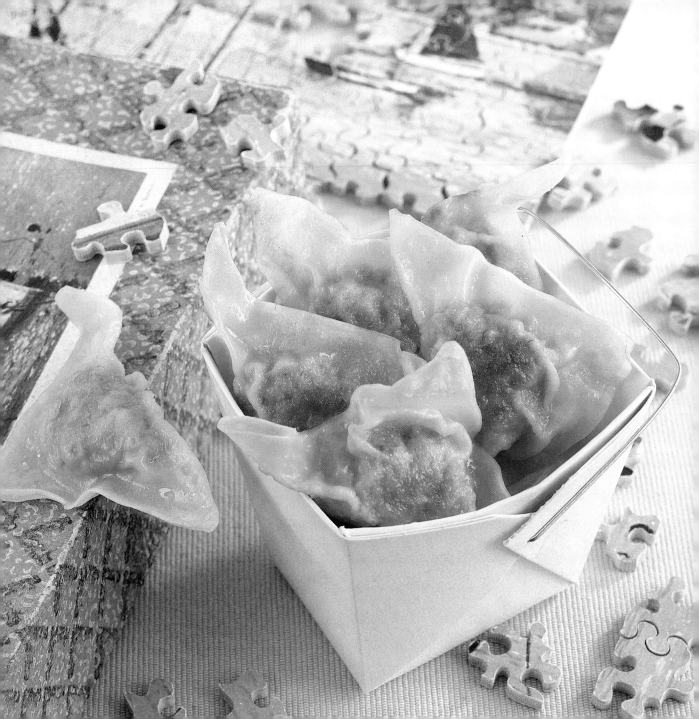

"Moneybag" Wontons

Wontons are great finger food and are surprisingly easy to make, plus children will enjoy helping to assemble the little packets. As you are working, keep the pile of wonton wrappers covered with damp paper towels and a piece of plastic wrap to stop them from drying out. You will also need a steamer basket and pan and some parchment paper.

Put 1 tablespoon of water in a medium saucepan and heat until steaming. Add the spinach, cover, and cook for 1 to 2 minutes, until the spinach has wilted. Drain and allow to cool slightly, then squeeze out as much liquid as possible.

Transfer the spinach to a food processor, add the shrimp and water chestnuts, and whiz briefly. Add the scallions, ginger, mirin, sugar, oyster sauce, and soy sauce, and pulse until the shrimp are roughly chopped.

Lay a wonton wrapper on a cutting board and dampen the edges. Put 2 teaspoonfuls of the filling in the center of the wonton and bring the corners together. Pinch just above the filling to seal. Alternatively, fold over to form a triangle. Set the wonton on a baking sheet lined with plastic wrap, and cover with another piece of plastic wrap. Repeat with the remaining wonton wrappers and filling.

The wontons can sit, covered, in the fridge for a couple of hours. If keeping any longer, follow the freezing instructions (right). To cook, line the base of a steamer basket with a circle of parchment paper (the Chinese often use lettuce leaves!) and place the wontons on top. Set the steamer over boiling water and cover. Steam the wontons for 8 minutes, or until cooked all the way through. Serve with extra soy sauce for dipping.

Preparation 25 minutes
Cook 8 minutes
Makes 12 wontons
Suitable for freezing: Put the covered wontons in the freezer for 2 to 3 hours, until solid. Transfer to a freezer bag and store in the freezer for up to 1 month. Steam directly from frozen, increasing the steaming time to 10 minutes. Not suitable for reheating.

1 cup packed baby spinach leaves, well washed
5 ounces raw large shrimp, peeled and deveined
4 or 5 water chestnuts, quartered
2 scallions, thinly sliced
½ teaspoon grated fresh ginger
1 teaspoon mirin
1 teaspoon sugar
1 teaspoon oyster sauce
½ teaspoon soy sauce, plus extra for dipping
12 wonton wrappers (available from Asian supermarkets in the refrigerator section)

TIP
If freezing, use shrimp that haven't been previously frozen, or use cooked shrimp.

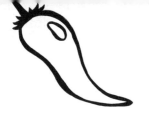

Sweet Chili Salmon Skewers

🥘 Preparation 5 minutes, plus marinating
🕐 Cook 7 minutes
🍽 Makes 4 skewers, 2 to 4 portions
❄ Not suitable for freezing or reheating

2 teaspoons sweet red chili sauce
1½ teaspoons mirin
½ teaspoon soy sauce
½ pound salmon fillet, skin removed, cut into ½-inch cubes

You will also need 4 wooden skewers, soaked in warm water for 30 minutes

Oily fish—for example, salmon—is a good source of omega-3 oils and should be offered a couple of times a week. Marinades, such as this delicious sweet red chili one, can help to tempt children who may not always want to try fish.

Mix the chili sauce, mirin, and soy sauce together in a bowl. Add the salmon and toss to coat. Set aside to marinate for 15 to 20 minutes, stirring two to three times.

Preheat the broiler and line a broiler pan with foil. Thread the salmon onto the skewers and set the skewers on the foil. Spoon over half of the marinade left in the bowl and broil the salmon for 3 minutes. Turn the skewers over, spoon over the rest of the marinade, and broil for 3 to 4 minutes more, until the salmon is cooked through.

Let cool slightly. For smaller children, it may be best to remove the salmon from the skewers before serving.

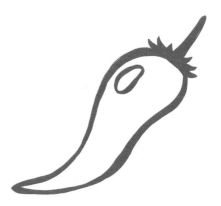

Teriyaki Salmon

You can vary this recipe, depending on your child's preferences. You could perhaps make it without the sesame seeds, and for children who aren't too keen on ginger, you may want to add just a little.

Preheat the broiler. Toast the sesame seeds by putting them in a small frying pan over medium heat for 2 to 3 minutes, stirring two or three times. Spread out on a plate and allow to cool.

Cut the salmon into ½-inch cubes. Thread 3 or 4 cubes onto each skewer and put the skewers on a foil-lined baking sheet.

Scrape the skin from the ginger using the tip of a teaspoon. Grate the ginger finely—you need ¼ teaspoon. Put the ginger in a bowl with the soy sauce and honey, and mix together.

Brush some of the sauce on the salmon and broil for 2 minutes, as close to the heat source as possible. Brush again with the sauce and broil for another 2 minutes. Turn the skewers over and repeat the brushing and broiling process.

Let the skewers cool slightly and serve sprinkled with the toasted sesame seeds. For smaller children, it may be a good idea to remove the salmon from the skewers before serving.

Preparation 5 minutes
Cook 8 minutes
Makes 6 skewers
Not suitable for freezing or reheating

1 tablespoon sesame seeds
7 ounces skinless salmon fillet
a small piece of fresh ginger
1½ teaspoons soy sauce
1 tablespoon honey

You will also need 6 wooden skewers, soaked in warm water for 30 minutes

TIP
It is easier to grate ginger if you freeze it first.

Pressed Sushi

⏱ Preparation 15 minutes
🕐 Cook 15 minutes
🌀 Makes about 32 sushi
❄ Not suitable for freezing
or reheating

1¼ cups sushi rice
1½ cups water
3 tablespoons rice vinegar
2 tablespoons sugar
¼ teaspoon salt
4 to 6 thin slices smoked salmon
 (about 5 ounces)
scallion strips and sesame seeds,
 for garnish (optional)
soy sauce, for dipping

TIP
This is a fun dish for older
children to make.

The Japanese call this type of sushi *oshi sushi,* and it is surprisingly easy to make. The sushi will cut more easily if you wet the knife between each cut. Although not suitable for freezing, it can be stored overnight in the fridge wrapped tightly in plastic wrap.

Put the rice in a saucepan with the water. Bring to a boil, cover the pan tightly, turn down the heat as low as possible, and cook for 15 minutes. Turn off the heat and let stand for another 15 minutes.

Meanwhile, warm the vinegar in a microwave for 10 seconds or warm gently in a saucepan, but do not boil, then stir in the sugar and salt until dissolved. Line an 8-inch springform pan with two pieces of plastic wrap, allowing plenty of overhang. Lay the smoked salmon on the base of the pan, overlapping the slices slightly.

Spoon the cooked rice into a large bowl and stir in the vinegar mixture. Let the rice cool for 10 minutes, stirring regularly. Spread the rice over the salmon, fold the plastic wrap over the top of the rice, then press the rice down firmly with a potato masher.

Chill for 30 minutes. Release the sides of the pan, unwrap the plastic wrap from the rice side, and flip the sushi disc onto a cutting board, salmon side up. Remove the plastic wrap and cut into pieces with a sharp knife. Garnish with scallion strips and sesame seeds if you like. Serve with soy sauce for dipping.

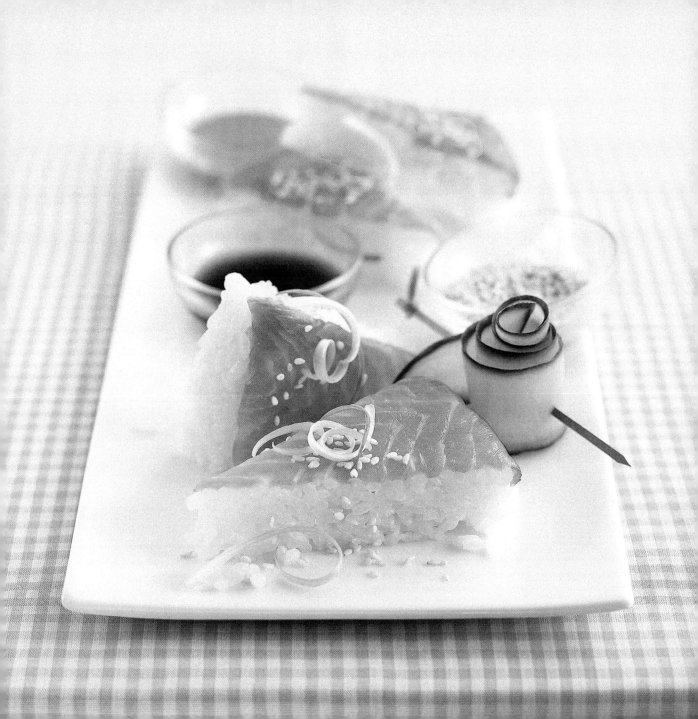

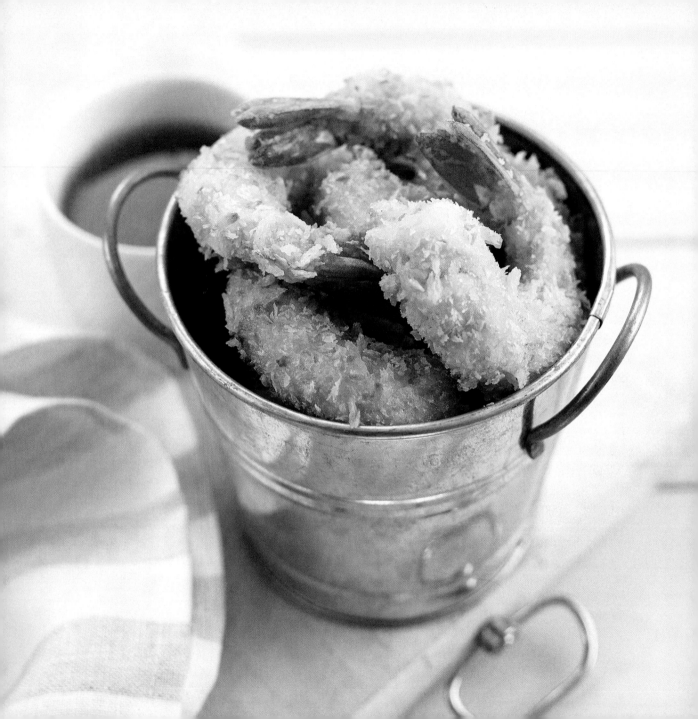

Coconut Shrimp

I'm not sure who thought of the addition of coconut originally, but the flavor seems to complement the sweetness of the shrimp. I love the very light and crispy Japanese panko bread crumbs, but if you can't find them, use regular unseasoned dried bread crumbs instead.

Mix the dipping sauce ingredients together in a small bowl. Divide among four smaller dipping bowls and set aside.

Pat the shrimp dry with paper towels. Spread out the flour on a large plate. Whisk the egg and soy sauce together in a bowl. Mix the bread crumbs and coconut together and spread out on a second plate. Dust the shrimp with the flour, then dip in the egg and roll in the coconut bread crumbs. Transfer to a plate or baking sheet. The crumb-coated shrimp can be kept in the fridge, covered, for up to 2 hours before cooking.

Put some canola oil in a wok or deep-sided frying pan, to the depth of 1/2 inch. Heat over medium heat until a bread cube dropped into the oil sizzles and browns in around 30 seconds. Add the shrimp and cook for 2 to 3 minutes on each side, until golden. If the shrimp are browning too quickly, lower the heat slightly. Don't overcrowd the pan—you may need to cook the shrimp in two batches. Drain the cooked shrimp on a couple of layers of paper towels and allow to cool slightly, then serve with the dipping sauce. The cocktail sauce from the Shrimp Cocktail Lettuce Boats (page 119) would make a good alternative dipping sauce.

Preparation 20 minutes, plus any thawing time
Cook 6 minutes
Makes 4 portions (recipe easily halved or doubled)
Not suitable for freezing or reheating

For the dipping sauce
2 tablespoons sweet red chili sauce
2 teaspoons rice vinegar
1 teaspoon mirin

12 large raw shrimp, peeled and deveined, tails on
2 tablespoons flour
1 egg
1/2 teaspoon soy sauce
1/3 cup panko bread crumbs, or 1/4 cup unseasoned dried bread crumbs
2 tablespoons unsweetened shredded coconut
canola oil, for frying

TIP
You can find unsweetened shredded coconut in health food stores.

Salmon Dip with Mock Melba Toast

Preparation 5 minutes plus chilling (dip), 5 minutes (toast)
Cook 8 minutes (for 4 pieces of toast)
Makes 4 portions
Not suitable for freezing or reheating

one 7.5-ounce can pink salmon, drained, with large pieces of skin and bone removed
2 ounces cream cheese
1 tablespoon ketchup
1 tablespoon mayonnaise
1 tablespoon Greek-style yogurt or sour cream
2 teaspoons fresh lemon juice
salt and pepper, to season
4 slices bread (whole-grain or white)

Canned salmon is a good source of calcium for growing children and making it into a dip can be a good way to tempt them to eat it. I love melba toast, but it is fiddly to prepare. This mock melba toast is quick to make and gives slices that are thin and crisp yet robust enough to survive dunking.

Put all the ingredients except the bread into a food processor with salt and pepper to taste. Pulse until well combined. Transfer to a bowl, cover, and chill for 1 to 2 hours (the dip will thicken slightly as it chills).

To make the toast, roll the bread with a rolling pin until thin. Cut off the crusts and toast the bread in a toaster (cut in half if slices are too large to fit into the toaster) or under the broiler for around 2 minutes, turning once, until golden and crisp. Cut into sticks, then lay on a wire cooling rack to help the toast crisp up further. Serve with the dip. The dip will keep, covered, in the fridge for 2 to 3 days.

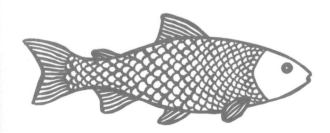

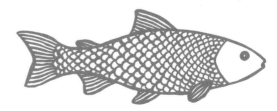

Smoked Salmon Rolls

The classic New York combination of salmon and cream cheese is beloved by adults and children alike. Toasted bagels are optional!

Put the cream cheese in a bowl and beat until softened. Mix in the lemon juice and dill or chives, if using, and season with pepper.

Lay out the salmon slices on a flat surface. You can make up the rolls in two ways: The cylinders have a solid cream cheese center; the pinwheels have "stripes." The rolls will keep, covered, in the fridge for 24 hours.

Cylinders

Put 1 tablespoon of the cream cheese mixture at one of the short ends of each slice of salmon and spread out slightly. Roll the slice of salmon up tightly from the cream cheese end to form a cylinder. If possible, cover and chill for 2 to 3 hours to allow the cream cheese to firm up. Cut into 4 slices.

Pinwheels

Spread 1 tablespoon of the cream cheese mixture over each slice of salmon. Roll up tightly from one of the short ends. If possible, cover and chill for 2 to 3 hours to allow the cream cheese to firm up. Cut into 5 slices.

🍳 Preparation 10 minutes, plus chilling
🍽 Makes 4 portions
☺ Not suitable for children under 1, as salt level is too high
❄ Suitable for freezing: Thaw overnight in the fridge.

2 ounces cream cheese (reduced-fat version or Neufchâtel is also fine)
½ teaspoon fresh lemon juice
½ teaspoon finely chopped fresh dill or snipped fresh chives (optional)
pepper, to season
4 large slices smoked salmon (about 4 ounces)

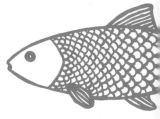

Finger-Licking Chicken

Chicken is popular with children and good for them, too—the dark meat contains twice as much iron and zinc as the white meat, supporting a healthy immune system and aiding growth and development. It's easy to make chicken nuggets—one of the most popular finger foods for children—and you can be sure they are good quality. Chicken on the grill is also delicious and ready in minutes. Take care, though: Chicken must be cooked thoroughly to prevent possible salmonella poisoning.

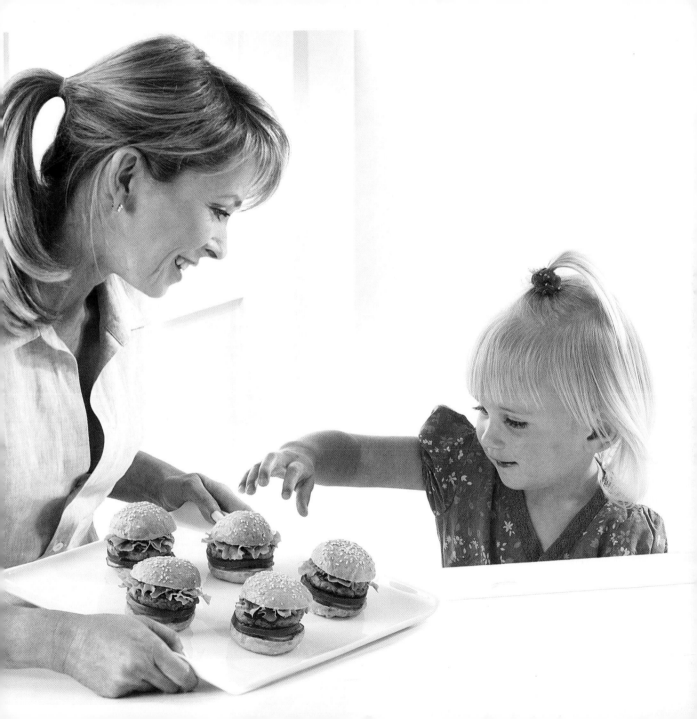

Parmesan Chicken Strips

🍲 Preparation 15 minutes
🕐 Cook 6 minutes
🍴 Makes 3 or 4 portions
☺ Suitable for children under 1
❄ Suitable for freezing: Put
the uncooked coated chicken
pieces on a baking sheet lined
with plastic wrap. Cover with a
second piece of plastic wrap and
freeze until firm, then transfer
to a freezer bag. Cook directly
from frozen, adding an extra
minute to the cooking time.
Not suitable for reheating
but good cold.

1 boneless, skinless chicken
   breast (about 5 ounces)
1 egg white
pepper, to season
½ cup freshly grated Parmesan

TIP
This is a good recipe for
children with wheat/gluten
allergies. Leftovers can be
used in the Mix 'n' Match
Pasta Salad (page 117).

Children seem to love the combination of cheese and chicken and may like to help making these easy chicken strips. You do need to make sure the chicken breast is beaten nice and thin, so that the chicken strips cook quickly. The chicken strips can be served warm with ketchup or my Quick Tomato Sauce (page 32), or cold in sandwiches with some mayonnaise and lettuce.

Cut the chicken breast in half horizontally through the center. Put the two pieces of chicken between two sheets of plastic wrap and beat with a mallet or rolling pin until ¼ inch thick. Remove the plastic wrap and cut the flattened chicken into small strips, about 2 inches long.

Beat the egg white with a little pepper until frothy. Spread the Parmesan out on a large plate. Dip the chicken strips in the egg white and roll in the Parmesan to coat.

Preheat the broiler and line a broiler pan with foil. Broil the chicken strips for 2 to 3 minutes, until the cheese is golden. Turn over and cook for 2 to 3 minutes more, until the chicken has cooked through. Let cool slightly before serving.

Cajun Chicken Skewers with Mango Salsa

You could also try making these using sweet smoked Spanish paprika, which is available in some supermarkets.

Preheat the broiler. Mix the chicken with the paprika, garlic, canola oil, and pepper. Thread the chicken onto 8 skewers. Place the chicken on a lightly oiled baking sheet and broil for 3 to 4 minutes on each side, until the chicken is cooked through.

To make the mango salsa, combine all the ingredients except the cilantro and seasoning, and set aside. Just before serving, add the cilantro and season well with salt and pepper.

For little ones, it is best to remove the chicken from the skewers before serving.

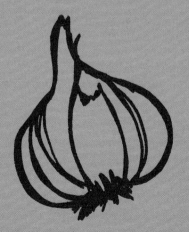

🍅 Preparation 5 minutes
🕐 Cook 8 minutes
🍽 Makes 8 skewers, 4 portions
❄ Not suitable for freezing or reheating

9 ounces boneless, skinless chicken breast, cut into strips
a pinch of paprika
1 or 2 garlic cloves, crushed
1 tablespoon canola oil
pepper, to season

You will also need 8 wooden skewers, soaked in warm water for 30 minutes

For the mango salsa
1/2 small red onion, very finely diced
1/2 ripe mango, very finely diced
1/2 teaspoon rice vinegar
juice of 1/2 lime
1 tablespoon chopped fresh cilantro
salt and pepper, to season

Chicken or Turkey Sliders

🍲 Preparation 15 minutes
🕐 Cook 24 minutes (assuming 3 batches)
🍪 Makes 22 sliders
❄ Suitable for freezing: Put tablespoonfuls of the mixture on a baking sheet lined with plastic wrap. Cover with more plastic wrap and freeze until solid, then transfer to a resealable container or freezer bag. Thaw overnight in the fridge and cook as directed. Not suitable for reheating.

3 slices white bread, crusts removed
¼ cup milk
1 red onion, finely chopped
1 tablespoon olive oil
1 garlic clove, crushed
9 ounces ground chicken or turkey
2 teaspoons soy sauce
3 tablespoons ketchup or tomato relish
1 teaspoon tomato paste
salt and pepper, to season
2 tablespoons canola oil, for frying

A slider is a bite-size burger. No one seems to be sure why they're called sliders—I can only assume it is because they slide down so easily when eaten! If you have older children, you could make these twice the size. Serve in the Baby Burger Buns (page 116). You can also serve these in mini buns with lettuce and ketchup or tomato relish.

Put the bread in a food processor and whiz to make bread crumbs. Add the milk.

Sauté the onion in the olive oil for 5 minutes, or until softened. Add the garlic and cook for a minute longer. Transfer to the food processor and add the remaining ingredients (seasoning to taste with the salt and pepper) except the canola oil. Whiz for 1 minute to chop and combine.

Heat the canola oil in a large frying pan. Drop the mixture by tablespoonfuls into the pan. Press down slightly using a wet teaspoon. Sauté for 2 to 3 minutes on each side, until golden and cooked through.

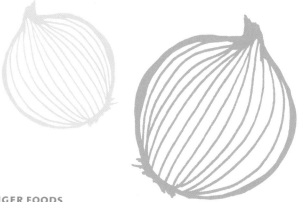

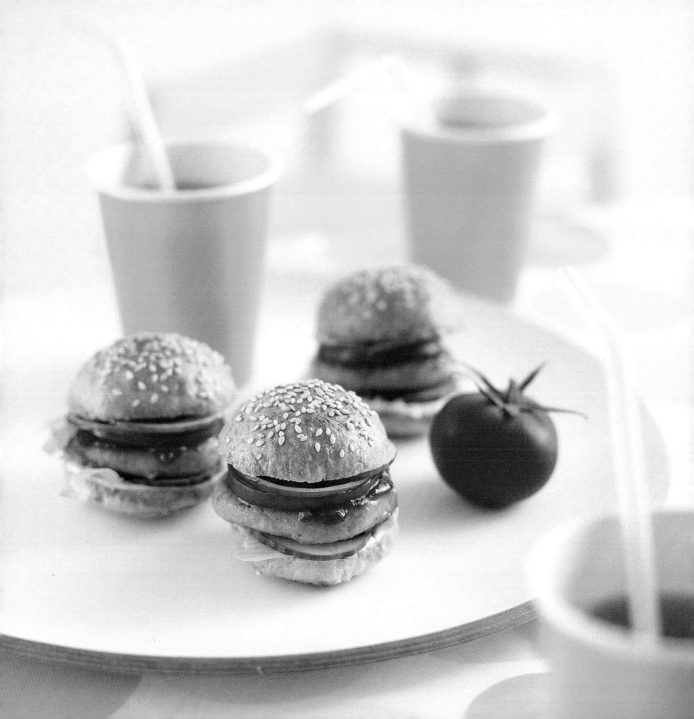

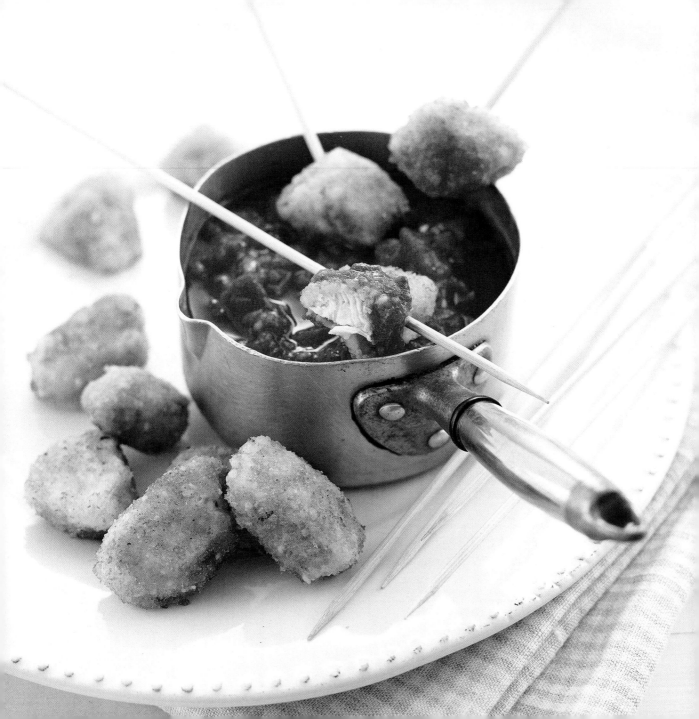

Krispie Chicken Nuggets

It will be hard to go back to store-bought nuggets after you have tasted these. You can skip the marinating stage if you don't have time, but it does add a delicious flavor to the chicken.

Cut the chicken into 1/2-inch cubes and put in a bowl. Mix together the 1/2 cup of milk, the garlic, thyme, lemon juice, 1/4 teaspoon salt, and some pepper (the mixture will separate a little from the lemon juice, but this is okay), and pour over the chicken. Cover and marinate in the fridge for at least 4 hours, or overnight.

Put the Rice Krispies in a food processor and whiz until reduced to fine crumbs. Add the cheeses plus salt and pepper to taste, and whiz to combine. Transfer to a large plate. Whisk the egg in a small bowl with the extra tablespoon of milk. Mix the flour with a little salt and pepper, and spread out on a large plate.

Remove the chicken pieces from the marinade, shaking off any excess. Toss in the seasoned flour, dip in the egg, and roll in the Rice Krispies coating. Put the oil in a large nonstick frying pan over medium heat. Fry the nuggets for 2 to 3 minutes on each side, until golden and crisp. Drain on paper towels and let cool slightly before serving.

Oven Method

Preheat the oven to 400°F. Reduce the oil to 2 tablespoons. Add 1 tablespoon oil to the Rice Krispies crumbs with the cheeses and whiz to combine evenly (you may need to stop and stir a couple of times). Grease a baking sheet with the remaining tablespoon of oil. Coat the chicken as above and put on the prepared baking sheet. Bake for 15 minutes, or until cooked through, turning over halfway.

Preparation 20 minutes, plus marinating
Cook 12 minutes
Makes 4 portions
Suitable for freezing: Put uncooked coated chicken on a baking sheet lined with plastic wrap. Cover with more plastic wrap, freeze until solid, then transfer to a freezer bag. Cook directly from frozen, adding 1 minute of extra cooking time for frying and 3 to 4 minutes for baking. Not suitable for reheating.

7 ounces boneless, skinless chicken breast
1/2 cup milk, plus 1 tablespoon
1 garlic clove, crushed
1 teaspoon fresh thyme leaves
1 tablespoon fresh lemon juice
salt and pepper, to season
1 1/2 cups Rice Krispies
2 tablespoons finely grated sharp Cheddar
1 tablespoon freshly grated Parmesan
1 egg
1/4 cup flour
3 to 4 tablespoons canola oil, for frying

TIP
Vary the marinade: Try 1/2 teaspoon dried oregano, and add paprika, cayenne, or Tabasco sauce if you like a bit of spice.

Sticky Soy Drumsticks

👐 Preparation 5 minutes,
plus marinating
🕐 Cook 35 to 40 minutes
🍳 Makes 6 drumsticks
❄ Suitable for freezing and
reheating. Uncooked drumsticks
can be frozen in their marinade
in a freezer bag. Thaw in the bag
overnight in the fridge and cook
as directed. Can be reheated for
30 seconds in a microwave only,
because otherwise they dry out
too much. However, they are
also good cold.

6 small skinless chicken
   drumsticks
2 tablespoons soy sauce
¼ cup fresh orange juice
1 teaspoon grated fresh ginger
1 garlic clove, crushed
2 tablespoons maple syrup

Kids tend to love drumsticks, and these are glazed with
a yummy combination of soy, ginger, and maple syrup. Just
remember to hand out wipes for those sticky fingers. I prefer
skinless drumsticks, to reduce the fat content, but you could
use skin-on.

Make a couple of cuts in the flesh of each drumstick and put the
drumsticks in a bowl or resealable freezer bag. Mix together the
soy sauce, orange juice, ginger, and garlic; pour over the chicken,
and stir or shake to cover the chicken in the marinade. Cover
or seal and marinate in the fridge for a minimum of 2 hours,
or overnight.

Preheat the oven to 400°F. Remove the drumsticks from the
marinade and set in a small baking dish that has been lined
with foil. Pour over the marinade left in the bowl or bag. Cover
the dish with foil and bake for 20 minutes.

Uncover the chicken, baste with the juices in the baking dish,
and drizzle with the maple syrup. Bake, uncovered, for 15 to
20 minutes more, basting every 5 minutes, until the drumsticks
are cooked through and coated in a sticky glaze.

The sugar in the glaze can be very hot, so it is a good idea
to allow the drumsticks to cool slightly before serving. Store
the cooked drumsticks in the fridge for up to 2 days.

Honey Dijon
Chicken Skewers

I love honey mustard, and this was the inspiration for the marinade. You can use whole-grain mustard instead if your children like spicier foods, but I find it has a little too much heat for smaller children.

Mix the honey, mustard, garlic, olive oil, and lemon juice together in a small bowl. Add the chicken and toss to coat, then cover and marinate overnight in the fridge.

Preheat the broiler and line a broiler pan with foil. Remove the chicken from the marinade and thread onto the skewers. Lay the skewers on the foil and spoon over any marinade left in the bowl. Broil for 3 to 4 minutes on each side, or until the chicken has cooked through.

Let cool slightly before serving. For smaller children, remove the chicken from the skewers and cut into bite-size chunks.

🍲 Preparation 5 minutes, plus marinating
🕐 Cook 8 minutes
🍴 Makes 4 skewers, 2 portions
❄ Suitable for freezing: You can freeze the chicken in the marinade in individual portion sizes. Thaw overnight in the fridge or in a microwave. Cook as directed. Not suitable for reheating, but these are also good cold.

1 tablespoon honey
1/2 teaspoon Dijon mustard
1/2 small garlic clove, crushed
1 teaspoon olive oil
1/2 teaspoon fresh lemon juice
4 chicken tenders (about
    1/4 pound total weight),
    or 1 small boneless, skinless
    chicken breast, sliced
    lengthwise into 4 strips, or
    into 3/4-inch cubes

You will also need 4 wooden
    skewers, soaked in warm
    water for 30 minutes.

Annabel's Chicken Croquettes

🍲 Preparation 20 minutes, includes 10 minutes for soaking the bread crumbs
🕐 Cook 21 minutes
🍥 Makes 12 croquettes
❄ Suitable for freezing

3 cups fresh bread crumbs, from white bread, crusts removed
4½ teaspoons milk
1 cup grated carrots
1 cup grated zucchini
2 tablespoons canola oil, for frying
1 medium onion, finely chopped
1 garlic clove, crushed
7 ounces ground chicken
1 teaspoon dried oregano
1 tablespoon ketchup
1½ teaspoons maple syrup
1 teaspoon soy sauce
½ teaspoon Worcestershire sauce
½ teaspoon balsamic vinegar
½ teaspoon sugar
salt and pepper, to season

For the coating
¼ cup flour
1 egg
3 to 4 tablespoons canola oil, for frying

You can sneak some vegetables into these tasty chicken croquettes. It is good to make a batch and freeze them on a baking sheet lined with plastic wrap. When frozen, wrap each one individually in plastic wrap so that you can take out just as many as you need.

Put a heaping cup of the bread crumbs into a bowl, add the milk, and let soak for 10 minutes. Squeeze a little of the moisture from the grated carrot and zucchini.

Heat the canola oil in a frying pan and sauté the onion for 3 minutes, stirring occasionally. Add the garlic and cook for 30 seconds, then add the carrot and zucchini, stirring for 5 minutes over low heat. Transfer to a plate and let cool.

Mix together the soaked bread, the chicken, cooked veggies, and remaining ingredients, seasoning to taste with the salt and pepper.

For the coating, spread out the flour on a large plate. Beat the egg in a small bowl. Using floured hands, form the mixture into patties, coat in the flour, dip in the egg, and coat with the remaining bread crumbs. Heat the oil in a frying pan and fry the croquettes, turning occasionally, for 12 minutes, or until golden brown. Drain on paper towels.

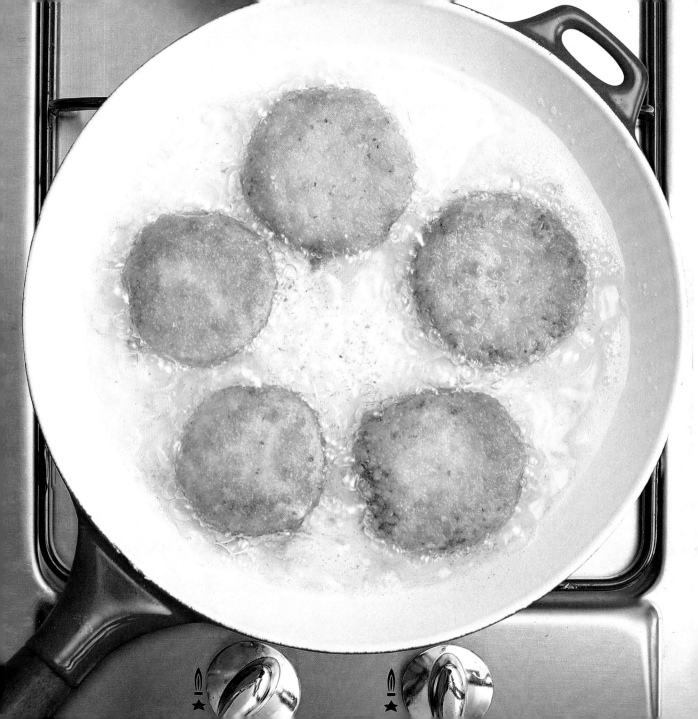

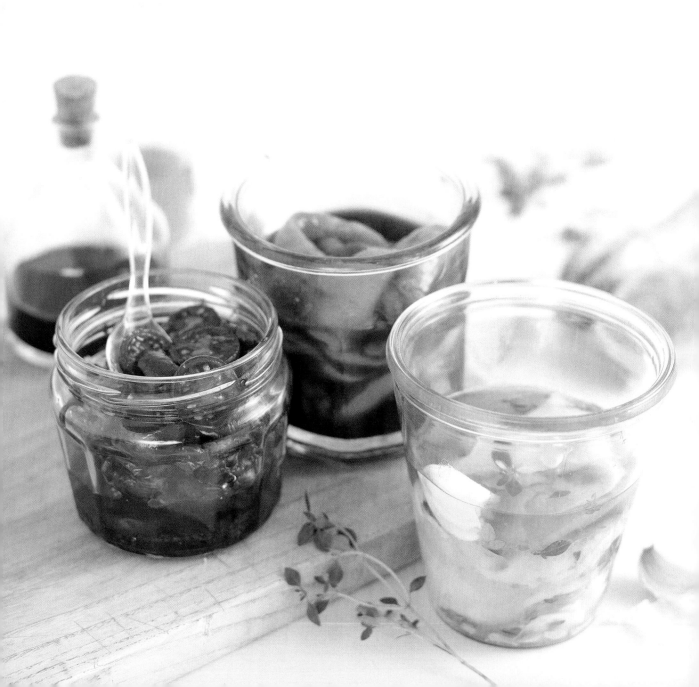

Marinated Chicken

Marinades not only add flavor but also tenderize chicken. You can marinate strips of uncooked chicken and freeze them so that they are ready to cook. This recipe is not suitable for reheating.

Preparation 5 to 10 minutes, plus marinating
Cook 8 minutes
Makes 4 skewers
Suitable for freezing

Tomato-Balsamic

Lemon & Thyme

Special Soy

For each marinade, mix together all the ingredients, transfer to a freezer bag or a bowl, and marinate the chicken in the fridge for at least 1 hour. While the chicken is marinating, soak 4 wooden skewers in warm water for 30 minutes. Season the chicken with salt and pepper before you cook it, but don't add the seasoning to the marinade.

If freezing the chicken, divide the chicken tenders into portions and put in small freezer bags. Divide the marinade among the bags, seal, and freeze. Thaw overnight in the fridge or in a microwave.

When you are ready to cook, preheat the broiler. Thread the chicken onto the skewers. Line a baking sheet with foil and broil the chicken tenders for 3 to 4 minutes on each side. Alternatively, you can cook them in a griddle pan. For smaller children, it is best to remove the chicken from the skewers before serving.

Tomato-Balsamic
3 cherry or grape tomatoes
2 small oil-packed sun-dried
  tomatoes, drained and chopped
2 tablespoons olive oil
$1\frac{1}{2}$ teaspoons balsamic vinegar
$\frac{1}{2}$ teaspoon light brown sugar
$\frac{1}{2}$ teaspoon tomato paste

Lemon & Thyme
$\frac{1}{4}$ teaspoon fresh thyme leaves
1 small garlic clove, crushed
2 tablespoons olive oil
2 teaspoons fresh lemon juice

Special Soy
$\frac{1}{4}$ teaspoon grated fresh ginger
1 teaspoon soy sauce
1 teaspoon rice vinegar
$\frac{1}{2}$ teaspoon tomato paste
$\frac{1}{2}$ teaspoon fresh lemon juice
$\frac{1}{2}$ teaspoon light brown sugar
1 tablespoon canola oil

$\frac{1}{4}$ pound chicken tenders or
  boneless, skinless chicken
  breast or thighs, cut into
  4 strips
salt and pepper, to season

BBQ Grilled Chicken

🍽 Preparation 5 to 10 minutes, plus marinating
🕐 Cook 8 minutes
🍳 Makes 2 to 4 portions
❄ Suitable for freezing. Not suitable for reheating.

For the marinade
2 tablespoons ketchup
1 tablespoon maple syrup
¼ teaspoon soy sauce
2 or 3 drops Worcestershire sauce

¼ pound chicken tenders or boneless, skinless chicken breast, cut into 4 strips
salt and pepper, to season

In the summer you can cook the marinated chicken on the barbecue. Personally, I prefer to use chicken on the bone for outdoor grilling, as it remains more moist. Just make sure that the chicken is thoroughly cooked. You can always strip the flesh from the bone before serving.

Mix together all the marinade ingredients in a freezer bag or a bowl and marinate the chicken in the fridge for at least 1 hour. Season the chicken with salt and pepper before you cook it, but don't add the seasoning to the marinade.

When you are ready to cook, preheat the broiler. Line a baking sheet with foil and broil the chicken tenders for 3 to 4 minutes on each side. Alternatively, you can cook the tenders on a griddle pan.

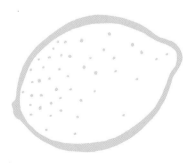

Chicken Tikka Skewers

Mild curry flavors can be popular with children. Feel free to use a stronger curry paste—but only if your children like spicy food!

Mix together in a bowl the yogurt, curry paste or powder, honey, and lemon juice. Add the chicken and stir to coat it in the marinade. Cover and marinate overnight in the fridge.

Preheat the broiler and line a broiler pan with foil. Remove the chicken from the marinade and thread onto the skewers. Lay the skewers on the foil and spoon over any marinade left in the bowl. Broil for 3 to 4 minutes on each side, or until the chicken has cooked through.

Let cool slightly before serving. For smaller children, remove the chicken from the skewers and cut into bite-size chunks.

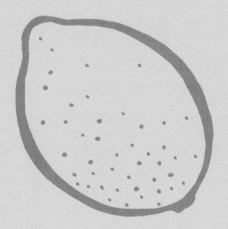

🍴 Preparation 5 minutes, plus marinating
🕐 Cook 8 minutes
🍳 Makes 4 skewers, 2 portions
❄ Suitable for freezing: Freeze the uncooked chicken in the marinade in individual portions. Thaw overnight in the fridge or in a microwave. Not suitable for reheating, but these are also good cold.

2 tablespoons Greek-style yogurt
1 teaspoon korma or mild curry paste (such as Patak's), or ½ teaspoon mild curry powder
½ teaspoon honey
½ teaspoon fresh lemon juice
¼ pound chicken tenders or boneless, skinless chicken breast, cut into 4 strips or 1½-inch cubes

You will also need 4 wooden skewers, soaked in warm water for 30 minutes

Chicken or Pork and Shrimp Dumplings

🍲 Preparation 15 minutes
🕐 Cook 8 minutes
🍽 Makes 10 dumplings
❄ Suitable for freezing: See method, right. Not suitable for reheating.

For the filling
5 ounces ground chicken
  or pork
¼ pound large raw shrimp,
  peeled, deveined, and
  roughly diced
1 large scallion, finely chopped
¼ teaspoon grated fresh ginger
1 tablespoon soy sauce
1 tablespoon sake
1 teaspoon Asian sesame oil
2 teaspoons cornstarch

10 wonton wrappers (available
  from Asian supermarkets)

For the dipping sauce
1 tablespoon soy sauce
1 tablespoon water
2 teaspoons rice vinegar
1 tablespoon light brown sugar
½ teaspoon Asian sesame oil
¼ teaspoon grated fresh ginger

peas, for garnish (optional)

My children always love going out with us for a Chinese meal, and they particularly like wontons and dim sum. These are not that difficult to make, and when I tested them for the first time, they were gobbled up by my three kids in less than 3 minutes.

Put the filling ingredients into a bowl and mix together.

Lay a wonton wrapper on a cutting board and dampen the edges. Put 2 teaspoonfuls of the filling in the center of the wonton and bring the corners toward each other, but don't actually seal together. Press the wonton gently onto the filling so it sticks to the filling and forms a round pouch shape but is still open in the center. Set the wonton on a baking sheet lined with plastic wrap, and cover with another piece of plastic wrap. Repeat with the remaining wonton wrappers and filling.

Oil the bottom of a bamboo or stainless-steel steamer and line with parchment paper. Remove the dumplings from the plastic wrap and put in the steamer, cover, and place over a saucepan of boiling water, making sure the water does not touch the base. Steam the dumplings for 6 to 8 minutes, until cooked.

To make the dipping sauce, stir all the ingredients together until the sugar has dissolved—if the sugar doesn't dissolve, warm gently in a saucepan over low heat.

Suitable for freezing: Freeze the uncooked plastic wrap–covered wontons for 2 to 3 hours, until solid. Transfer to a freezer bag and store in the freezer for up to 1 month. Steam directly from frozen, increasing the steaming time by 5 to 6 minutes, until cooked through. Garnish with peas, if desired.

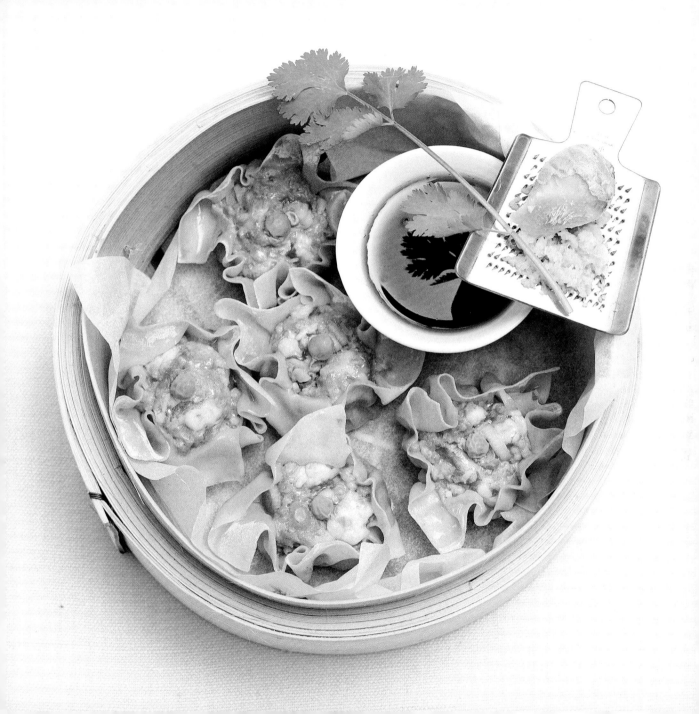

Chinese Glazed Chicken Wings

🍲 Preparation 5 minutes
🕐 Cook 35 minutes
🍳 Makes 3 or 4 portions
❄ Suitable for freezing: The uncooked chicken wings can be frozen in their marinade. Thaw thoroughly overnight in the fridge and cook as directed. Not suitable for reheating.

1 garlic clove, crushed
½ teaspoon grated fresh ginger
1 shallot, finely chopped
2 tablespoons oyster sauce
2 tablespoons soy sauce
1 teaspoon rice vinegar
1 tablespoon honey
6 chicken wings, wing tips removed, cut in half at the joint

There is something quite irresistible about sweet and sticky chicken, and my easy Chinese wings are no exception. In the unlikely event of leftovers, they are also very good served cold.

Mix all of the ingredients except the chicken together in a large bowl. Add the chicken wings and toss to coat. Cover and marinate in the fridge overnight, turning the chicken wings once in the marinade (you can also marinate the wings in a large, resealable freezer bag).

Preheat the oven to 400°F. Line a small baking dish with foil. Pour the wings and their marinade into the dish and cover with a second sheet of foil. Roast for 20 minutes, then uncover and roast for 10 to 15 minutes more, turning every 5 minutes, until the chicken wings are shiny, sticky, and cooked through.

Let cool before serving—the sticky glaze can be very hot when first out of the oven. Leftovers can be kept in the fridge for up to 2 days.

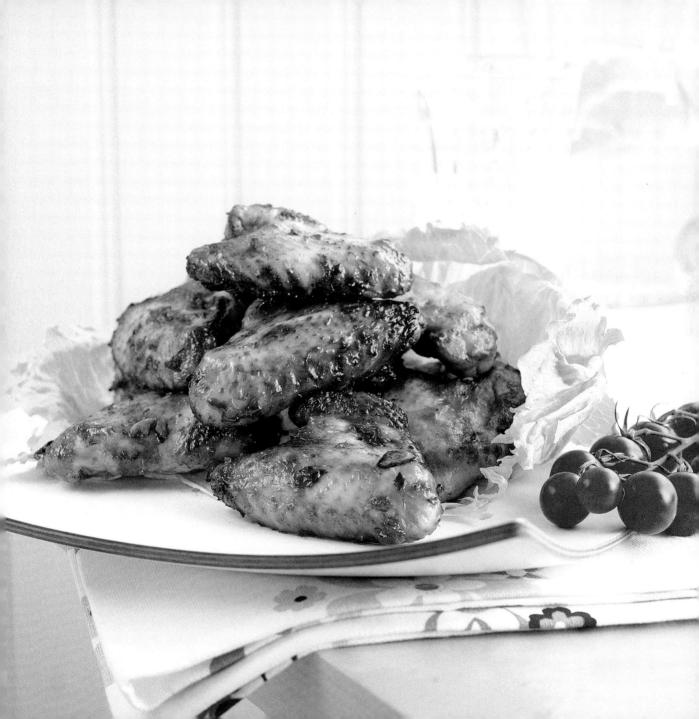

Mini Chicken Sausages

🍽 Preparation 10 minutes
🕐 Cook 6 minutes
🍳 Makes 6 sausages
☺ Suitable for children under 1 year old
❄ Not suitable for reheating

½ small red onion, diced
1 tablespoon olive oil
2 tablespoons fresh bread crumbs, from ½ slice white bread, crusts removed
5 ounces ground chicken
½ large apple, peeled and grated
1 teaspoon chopped fresh parsley
2 tablespoons freshly grated Parmesan
½ chicken bouillon cube, dissolved in 1½ teaspoons boiling water
1 tablespoon flour
3 or 4 tablespoons canola oil, for frying

The combination of grated apple, sautéed red onion, and Parmesan cheese gives these little sausages a lovely flavor. They are good hot or cold, and are just the right size for small fingers.

Sauté the onion in the olive oil for 5 minutes. Transfer to a food processor with the bread crumbs, chicken, apple, parsley, Parmesan, and bouillon, and whiz to combine. Roll tablespoonfuls into sausage shapes and chill for 1 hour.

Put the flour on a large plate and dust the sausages with flour. Heat the canola oil in a frying pan and fry the sausages for 5 to 6 minutes on medium heat, turning frequently, until golden. Drain on paper towels before serving.

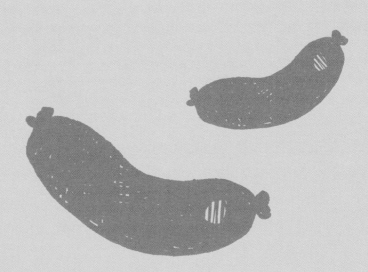

Satay Chicken Skewers

Chicken tenders are useful, as they are ready-portioned, but it is easy to cut up a chicken breast if that is all you have. I tend not to serve the dip to smaller children—it is so yummy that they just scoop it up and eat it neat, rather than dipping the chicken in it.

Mix the ginger, garlic, lime juice, soy sauce, honey, and peanut butter together in a medium bowl. Add the chicken and toss to coat. Cover and marinate for a minimum of 30 minutes, or overnight in the fridge.

Preheat the broiler and line a broiler pan with foil. Remove the chicken from the marinade and thread 1 piece onto each skewer. Lay the skewers on the foil and spoon over any marinade left in the bowl. Broil for 3 to 4 minutes on each side, until the chicken has cooked through.

If making the satay dip, put all of the ingredients into a small saucepan and melt together over low heat, stirring constantly. Bring to a boil and cook for around 1 minute, until thickened. Remove from the heat and let cool to room temperature before serving.

Serve the chicken skewers with the dip. For smaller children, remove the chicken from the skewers and cut into bite-size chunks.

Preparation 5 minutes, plus marinating
Cook 9 minutes
Makes 4 skewers, 2 portions
Suitable for freezing: Freeze the uncooked chicken in the marinade in individual portions. Thaw overnight in the fridge or in a microwave. Not suitable for reheating, but also good cold.

1/2 teaspoon grated fresh ginger
1/2 garlic clove, crushed
2 teaspoons fresh lime juice
2 teaspoons soy sauce
2 teaspoons honey
4 teaspoons peanut butter
4 chicken tenders (about 1/4 pound total weight), or 1/4 pound boneless, skinless chicken breast or thighs, cut into 4 strips

You will also need 4 wooden skewers, soaked in warm water for 30 minutes

For the satay dip (optional)
3 tablespoons creamy peanut butter
3 tablespoons coconut milk
2 tablespoons water
2 teaspoons sweet red chili sauce
1/2 teaspoon soy sauce

Apricot-Dijon Drumsticks

🍲 Preparation 5 minutes,
plus marinating
🕐 Cook 30 to 35 minutes
🎂 Makes 6 drumsticks
❄ Suitable for freezing and
reheating. The uncooked
drumsticks can be frozen in
the marinade in a freezer bag.
Thaw overnight in the fridge
and cook as directed. Reheat
cooked drumsticks for 30
seconds in the microwave only,
otherwise the drumsticks
become too dry.

3 tablespoons apricot jam
2 teaspoons Dijon mustard
1 teaspoon fresh lemon juice
6 skinless chicken drumsticks
   (about 1¼ pounds total
   weight), or skin-on, if
   you prefer
salt and pepper, to season

Fruit and mustard may be a slightly unusual combination, but it is a delicious mix of sweet and piquant that should appeal to all the family.

Mix together the jam, mustard, and lemon juice in a small bowl. Make two or three cuts in the flesh of each drumstick and put the drumsticks in a large bowl or resealable freezer bag. Pour the marinade over the drumsticks and toss to coat. Cover or seal and marinate in the fridge for at least 4 hours or overnight.

Preheat the oven to 400°F. Put the drumsticks in a baking dish lined with foil and season with salt and pepper. Pour over the marinade left in the bag, cover with foil, and bake the drumsticks for 20 minutes. Uncover, turn over the drumsticks, and baste with the juices in the pan. Cook, uncovered, for 10 to 15 minutes more, basting every 5 minutes with the juices in the pan, until the chicken has cooked through. Let cool slightly before serving and serve warm; they are also good cold. The cooked drumsticks will keep in the fridge for 2 to 3 days.

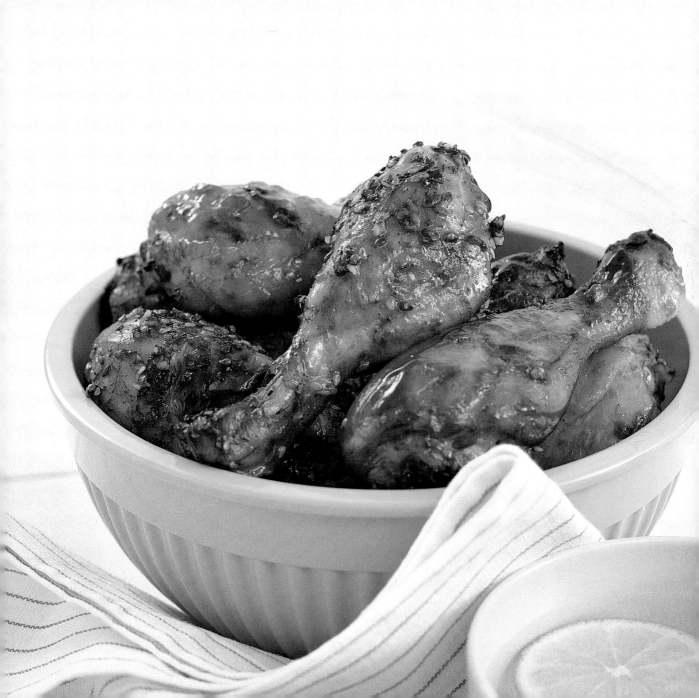

Cheat's Spring Rolls

🍲 Preparation 5 minutes
🕐 Cook 7 minutes
🍥 Makes 2 portions
❄ Not suitable for freezing
or reheating

1 tablespoon canola oil
¼ pound boneless, skinless
   chicken breast, cut into
   very small strips
1 small carrot, coarsely grated
a handful of bean sprouts
1 scallion, thinly sliced
½ teaspoon soy sauce
1 tablespoon plum sauce
two 7-inch flour tortillas

TIP
If the rolls won't stay shut,
secure with a toothpick
when you turn them over.
Remove the toothpick
before serving.

Chinese spring rolls are so yummy, but as they are deep-fried, they are a bit unhealthy—and tricky to do at home. So I came up with this healthy and easy-to-make version that is just as crispy and delicious.

Preheat the broiler. Heat the oil in a wok or large frying pan and stir-fry the chicken for 2 minutes. Add the vegetables and stir-fry for 2 minutes more, or until the chicken has cooked through and the vegetables have softened slightly (but aren't completely soft). Stir in the soy sauce and 1 teaspoon of the plum sauce, and remove from the heat.

Spread the remaining plum sauce over the tortillas (a teaspoon on each). Divide the filling between the tortillas, spooning it onto the lower half of each tortilla. Fold over the left- and right-hand sides of the tortilla, then roll up from the bottom, so that the filling is completely enclosed.

Carefully transfer the filled tortillas to a broiler pan, setting them seam side down. Broil for 1 to 1½ minutes, until the tops are crisp and starting to brown, then turn over and broil for 1 to 1½ minutes more. Watch carefully, as the tortillas can scorch easily. Serve immediately.

Buffalo Wings

The name Buffalo wings comes from the city of Buffalo in New York State, where they were first served. They are usually very spicy, but this is my child-friendly version, which is still finger-licking good!

Preheat the oven to 400°F.

Cut off the tips of the chicken wings and discard. Cut the remaining part of the wings into two at the joint and put on a baking sheet. Season with salt, pepper, and a little paprika, and bake for 40 to 45 minutes, until golden and crisp. Alternatively, you can broil or grill the wings for 20 to 30 minutes, turning frequently.

Meanwhile, put the ketchup, broth, butter, and chili sauce in a small saucepan. Heat gently, stirring, until the butter has melted, then remove from the heat.

Transfer the cooked wings to a large bowl, pour over the sauce, and toss to coat the wings. Return the wings to their baking sheet and bake for 5 to 7 minutes more, until glazed, or broil/grill for an extra 2 to 3 minutes. Serve immediately.

Preparation 10 minutes
Cook 52 minutes
Makes 3 or 4 portions
Not suitable for freezing. Leftovers are unlikely, but the cooled wings will keep in the fridge for up to 2 days. Not suitable for reheating, but just as tasty served cold!

6 whole chicken wings
salt, pepper, and paprika, to season
¼ cup ketchup
3 tablespoons vegetable broth
1 tablespoon butter
1 or 2 teaspoons sweet red chili sauce (or to taste)

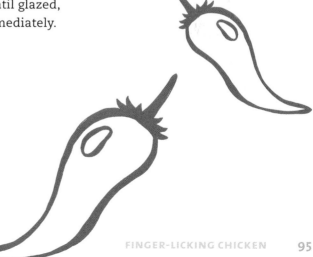

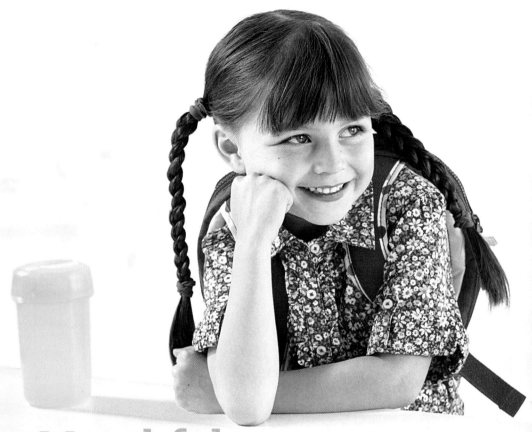

Meaty Mouthfuls

I find ground meat tends to be more popular with younger children than chunks of meat, as they often don't like chewing on something hard. It is really important to include meat in your child's diet, as it's a good source of iron. The most common nutritional deficiency in young children is iron deficiency, which leads to fatigue, lack of concentration, and impaired mental and physical development.

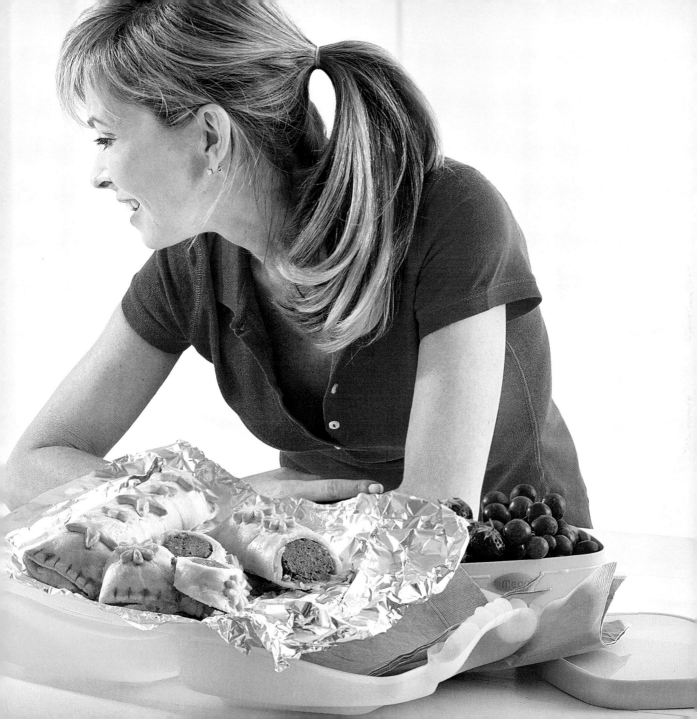

Meatballs in BBQ Sauce

⊛ Preparation 20 minutes
🕐 Cook 40 minutes
⊛ Makes about 25 meatballs
❄ Suitable for freezing: Freeze cooked meatballs in their sauce. Thaw overnight in the fridge. Reheat in a microwave for 30 seconds to 1 minute. (Timing will depend on the quantity of meatballs.) Or heat in a saucepan for about 5 minutes, adding a splash of water if the sauce becomes too thick.

1 medium red onion, finely chopped
1 tablespoon olive oil
3 fresh thyme sprigs
1 cup fresh bread crumbs, from about 3 slices white bread, crusts removed
9 ounces ground beef
2 tablespoons milk
1 teaspoon honey
salt and pepper, to season

For the BBQ sauce
scant ½ cup ketchup
⅔ cup fresh orange juice
2 tablespoons honey
2 tablespoons soy sauce
3 tablespoons water
1 garlic clove, crushed

Meatballs are always popular with small children, as they are tender and easy to chew. This BBQ sauce makes a delicious change from the usual tomato sauce.

Preheat the oven to 400°F.

Sauté the onion in the oil for 5 to 6 minutes, or until soft. Pick the leaves from the thyme (you should have ¼ teaspoon) and put in a large bowl. Add the sautéed onion, bread crumbs, ground beef, milk, and honey, and season with salt and pepper to taste.

Mix together with your hands until thoroughly combined. Roll teaspoonfuls of the mixture into about 25 small balls. Put in a lightly oiled large baking dish. Bake for 15 minutes.

Mix together all the ingredients for the sauce, pour over the meatballs, and bake for 20 to 25 minutes more, stirring gently once or twice. Serve with rice.

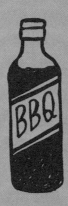
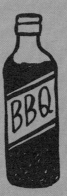
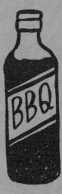

Maple-Ginger
Sticky Sausages

Sticky sausages are a perennial British favorite, and I have updated the traditional honey mixture by using maple syrup and a dash of fresh ginger. These are yummy warm or cold—and don't forget wet wipes to clean fingers and faces.

Preheat the oven to 400°F.

Put the sausages into a small baking dish, lined with foil for easier cleanup. Bake for 10 minutes. Meanwhile, mix together the maple syrup, soy sauce, and ginger.

Spoon off any excess fat from the baking dish. Pour the maple mixture over the sausages and stir so that the sausages are coated in the glaze. Bake for 25 minutes more, stirring every 10 minutes and keeping a close eye on the sausages in the last 5 minutes.

Transfer the sausages to a plate or bowl and allow to cool for around 10 minutes before serving—the glaze can be quite hot, so check the temperature before serving to smaller children. Leftovers can be kept in the fridge, covered, for up to 2 days.

Preparation 5 minutes
Cook 35 minutes
Makes 12 small sausages, 4 to 6 portions
Not suitable for freezing or reheating, but nice cold

12 skinny breakfast sausage links
3 tablespoons maple syrup
1 tablespoon soy sauce
1/2 teaspoon grated fresh ginger

Italian-Style
Mini Meatballs

🍲 Preparation 40 minutes
🕐 Cook 30 minutes, plus 2 to
3 minutes for cheesy topping
🥧 Makes about 30 meatballs
☺ Suitable for children under 1
❄ Suitable for freezing and
reheating: Brown the meatballs,
cool, and mix with the sauce.
Freeze in portions. Thaw in the
fridge. Reheat gently in a pan
or bake for 25 minutes at 400°F.

For the sauce
1 tablespoon olive oil
1 medium red onion, chopped
1 garlic clove, crushed
one 14-ounce can diced
    tomatoes
4¹/₂ teaspoons tomato paste
1 tablespoon ketchup
1 teaspoon light brown sugar
¹/₄ teaspoon dried oregano
¹/₄ cup vegetable broth

¹/₄ pound ground beef
¹/₄ pound ground veal
¹/₄ pound ground pork
¹/₃ cup fresh white bread crumbs
3 tablespoons milk
a small handful of parsley
    leaves, chopped
(Continued on page 102)

These are perfect for small mouths. You could substitute ground chicken for either the veal or pork, or use just one type of ground meat.

First make the sauce. Heat the oil in a large pan and sauté the onion for 10 minutes, or until soft. Add the garlic, cook for 1 minute, then transfer half to a food processor. Add the tomatoes, tomato paste, ketchup, sugar, oregano, and vegetable broth to the onions left in the pan, bring to a boil, reduce the heat, and simmer for 25 minutes.

Meanwhile, add the ground beef, veal, and pork to the onion in the food processor. Whiz for a minute to chop everything, then add the bread crumbs, milk, parsley, and Parmesan, seasoning with salt and pepper to taste. Pulse until well combined. Form rounded teaspoonfuls of the meatball mixture into about 30 small balls. You can now either fry the meatballs or bake them in the oven.

For frying: Heat the canola oil in a large nonstick frying pan and fry in batches of 8 to 10 meatballs for 2 to 3 minutes on each side, until golden. Drain on paper towels.

For oven browning: Preheat the oven to 400°F. Put a baking sheet in the oven when you turn it on and allow it to heat up. Put 2 tablespoons of canola oil on the hot baking sheet and add the meatballs. Bake for 20 minutes, turning halfway through.

Puree the sauce until smooth, and season to taste with salt and pepper. Return to the saucepan and add the browned meatballs, using a slotted spoon. Simmer for 5 to 10 minutes more. Serve with spaghetti or in hollowed-out French bread.

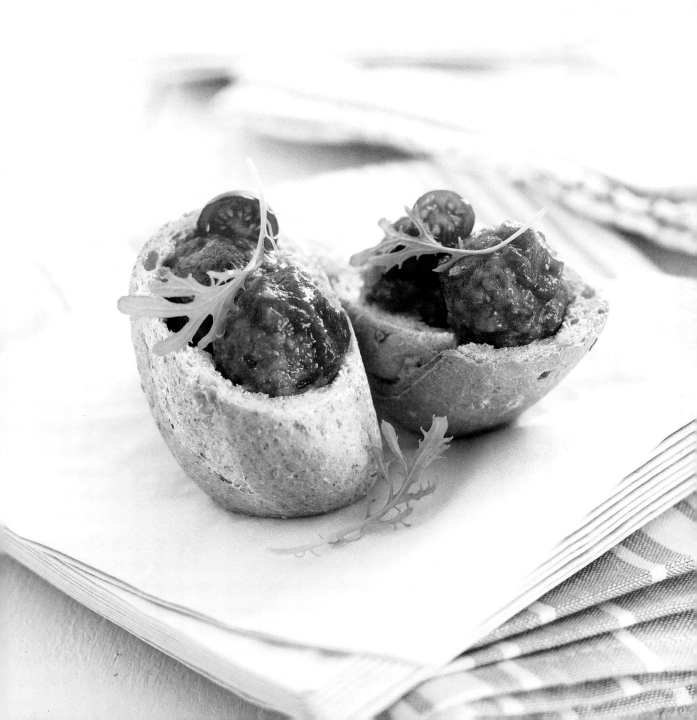

(Continued from page 100)
2 tablespoons freshly grated
   Parmesan
salt and pepper, to season
2 or 3 tablespoons canola oil,
   for frying

Optional Cheesy Topping

Transfer the cooked meatballs and sauce to a baking dish, sprinkle with 1 cup grated Cheddar or mozzarella, and pop under a preheated broiler for 2 to 3 minutes, until the cheese is golden and bubbling.

Sloppy Joe Pitas

🍲 Preparation 5 minutes
🕐 Cook 15 minutes
🍽 Makes 2 portions
❄ Suitable for freezing and reheating. Leftover sauce can be frozen for up to 1 month. Reheat in a microwave for 1 to 2 minutes, or for 5 minutes in a small pan over medium heat.

1¹/2 teaspoons olive oil
¹/2 small onion, finely chopped
¹/2 medium carrot, grated
   (optional)
¹/2 small garlic clove, crushed
¹/4 pound ground beef (you can
   also use chicken or turkey)
scant ¹/2 cup tomato sauce
2 teaspoons ketchup
2 small pitas, or 1 large pita,
   halved crosswise

A sloppy joe is typically served in a burger bun. I prefer to serve it in pita bread, as there is slightly less chance of the filling leaking out. Either way it is delicious—if a little messy at times!

Heat the oil in a wok or medium frying pan and sauté the onion and carrot, if using, for 4 minutes, or until soft. Add the garlic and ground beef, and continue to sauté for 5 minutes more, or until the beef is browned. Keep stirring regularly to break the meat into small pieces.

Add the tomato sauce and ketchup, and simmer briskly for 4 to 5 minutes, until most of the liquid has evaporated and the sauce is nice and thick. Meanwhile, warm the pitas for a few seconds in a microwave, then carefully slice open to make pockets. Spoon the sloppy joe mixture into the pitas (don't overfill) and serve warm. Any leftover sauce can be kept in the fridge, covered, for up to 2 days.

Finger-Sized Mini Meat Loaves

Rather than making a large meat loaf and slicing, I sometimes like to make these finger-sized ones so little eaters feel they have something special of their own. Pop one into a Baby Burger Bun (page 116) for a mini meat loaf sandwich!

Preheat the oven to 400°F. Generously oil 16 cups in two 12-cup mini muffin pans.

Mix the ketchup, sugar, and Worcestershire sauce together in a small bowl, and set aside (if the sugar won't dissolve, warm the mixture for 10 to 20 seconds in a microwave or gently for a few minutes in a saucepan over low heat).

Put the bread crumbs and milk in a large bowl and let soak for 5 minutes. Meanwhile, sauté the onion and garlic in the olive oil for 5 minutes. Add the sautéed onion to the bread crumbs, along with the beef, thyme, and 2 tablespoons of the ketchup mixture. Season to taste with salt and pepper, and mix together (for a finer texture, pulse in a food processor).

Divide the mixture among 16 cups in the muffin pans (approximately 1 tablespoon each). Brush half of the remaining ketchup mixture over the tops of the meat loaves and bake for 15 minutes. Brush again with the remaining ketchup mixture and bake for 15 minutes more. Remove from the oven and let stand for 10 minutes (they need standing time to firm up a bit). Run a knife around the edge of each meat loaf and ease it out of the pan with a teaspoon. Serve warm or cold. Any leftovers will keep in the fridge for up to 2 days.

Preparation 15 minutes
Cook 30 minutes
Makes approximately 16 meat loaves, 4 to 8 portions
Suitable for freezing: Cooked meat loaves can be frozen. Suitable for reheating, preferably for 10 to 15 seconds in a microwave; otherwise wrap in foil and reheat at 350°F for 10 to 15 minutes.

5 tablespoons ketchup
1 tablespoon light brown sugar
1/4 teaspoon Worcestershire sauce
2/3 cup fresh bread crumbs, from 2 slices white bread, crusts removed
1/3 cup milk
1 small red onion, grated
1 garlic clove, crushed
2 teaspoons olive oil
1/2 pound ground beef
1/2 teaspoon chopped fresh thyme, or 1/4 teaspoon dried thyme
salt and pepper, to season

Chinese BBQ Ribs

🍲 Preparation 5 minutes,
plus marinating
🕐 Cook 1¼ hours
🍽 Makes 4 portions
❄ Suitable for freezing: The
uncooked ribs can be frozen in
the marinade. Thaw overnight
in the fridge, then bake as
directed. Reheating is not
ideal, but you can reheat in a
microwave for around a minute
on high or wrapped in foil in the
oven at 350°F for 20 minutes.

⅓ cup fresh orange juice
¼ cup ketchup
3 tablespoons plum sauce
4½ teaspoons hoisin sauce
4½ teaspoons light brown
    sugar
2 pounds St. Louis–style ribs, cut
    into individual ribs (about 12)

TIP
I like to marinate the ribs
overnight, as it allows the
flavor to penetrate, but if you
don't have time, you can just
toss the ribs in the sauce and
bake immediately.

Spareribs are easy for children to hold and are usually very
popular. Hoisin sauce is often known as "Chinese barbecue
sauce," and it is a common ingredient in *char siu*—Chinese roast
pork. The marinade is also delicious for chicken wings.

Mix together the liquid ingredients and sugar in a large bowl
or resealable plastic bag to make the marinade. Add the ribs
and toss to coat. Cover the bowl or seal the bag, and marinate
overnight in the fridge.

Preheat the oven to 350°F and line a small roasting pan
with foil. Set the ribs in the prepared pan and pour over the
marinade from the bowl or bag. Cover the pan with a second
piece of foil and bake the ribs for 30 minutes. Uncover and bake
for 30 minutes more. Turn the oven up to 400°F and bake for
another 10 to 15 minutes, turning halfway through, until the
ribs are glazed and sticky.

Transfer to a plate and allow the ribs to cool slightly before
serving. Check the temperature before serving—the marinade
can get very hot and takes a while to cool down.

Beef Skewers with Balsamic–Brown Sugar Glaze

Skewers make perfect finger food, as the pieces of meat are cut into bite-size portions and the skewer makes a great vehicle for older children to eat from. This sweet and tangy glaze works very well with beef. Smaller children, though, may find even beef tenderloin a little too chewy—so you can always make these skewers with chicken instead.

Put the balsamic vinegar, sugar, and water in a small saucepan over medium heat. Bring to a boil, stirring constantly, then lower the heat and simmer for 2 to 3 minutes, until reduced by half and looking syrupy (the glaze will leave a light coating on the bottom of the pan if you tip it slightly).

Pour into a bowl and let cool for 5 minutes. Add the beef and toss to coat. Marinate for 10 to 15 minutes.

Preheat the broiler and line a broiler pan with foil. Slide the beef cubes onto the skewers and set them on the foil-lined pan. Spoon over half of the marinade left in the bowl. Broil for 3 to 4 minutes. Turn the skewers over, spoon on the remaining marinade, and broil for 3 to 4 minutes more, until the beef has cooked through.

Transfer the skewers to a plate and spoon on any juices sitting on the foil. Let cool slightly before serving. For smaller children, it may be better to remove the beef from the skewers before serving. Any leftovers will keep in the fridge, covered, for up to 2 days.

Preparation 5 minutes, plus 15 minutes' marinating
Cook 8 minutes
Makes 4 skewers, 2 portions
Not suitable for freezing. Suitable for reheating in a microwave for 1 minute (remove skewers first).

2 tablespoons balsamic vinegar
4¹⁄₂ teaspoons light brown sugar
1 tablespoon water
5 ounces beef tenderloin or trimmed strip steak, cut into ¹⁄₂-inch cubes

You will also need 4 wooden skewers, soaked in warm water for 30 minutes

TIP
Don't be tempted to marinate the meat for too long—the vinegar is acidic and will break down the meat proteins quickly, which means the meat will turn mushy.

Mini Bacon and Egg Tarts

🍲 Preparation 25 minutes
🕐 Cook 17 minutes
🍴 Makes 12 tarts
❄️ Suitable for freezing: Freeze the cooked tarts. Thaw overnight in the fridge. Suitable for reheating in a microwave for about 10 seconds or in an oven at 350°F for 10 minutes.

one 7.5-ounce store-bought refrigerated piecrust
2 ounces thinly sliced bacon (about 2 slices)
1 teaspoon olive oil
5 tablespoons milk
1 tablespoon heavy cream (or use 6 tablespoons milk)
1 egg plus 1 extra yolk
pepper, to season

Kids tend to love things with bacon, and these mini tarts—manageable for small hands—are no exception. Serve them warm with salad and also cold for lunch boxes or picnics.

Roll out the piecrust to 1/16 inch thick. Cut out circles using a 2¼-inch round cookie cutter. Gather up and reroll the pastry trimmings, if needed, until you have 12 pastry circles. Gently ease the pastry circles into the cups of a mini muffin pan. Chill for 15 minutes.

Meanwhile, preheat the oven to 400°F.

Cut the bacon into small pieces and sauté in the oil for 5 to 6 minutes, until crisp. Drain briefly on paper towels and divide the bacon among the pastry cups. Whisk together the milk, cream or extra milk, egg, and egg yolk and season with a little pepper (no salt, as the bacon is salty enough). Pour the egg mixture into the pastry cups, filling almost to the top.

Bake for 15 to 17 minutes, until slightly puffed and golden around the edges. Remove from the oven and let stand for 5 to 10 minutes before removing the tarts from the pan (run a sharp knife around the edge of each tart to help release it). Serve warm or refrigerate in a resealable container as soon as cool. Leftovers can be kept in the fridge for up to 2 days.

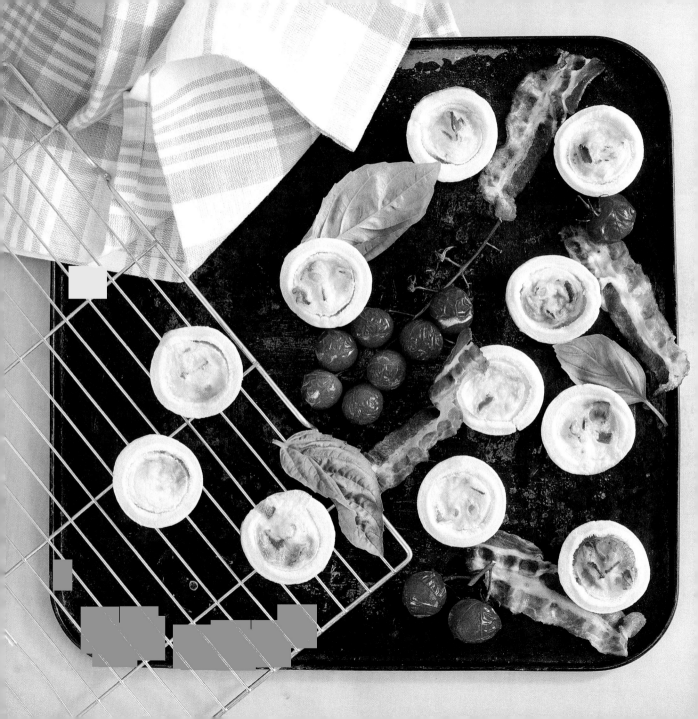

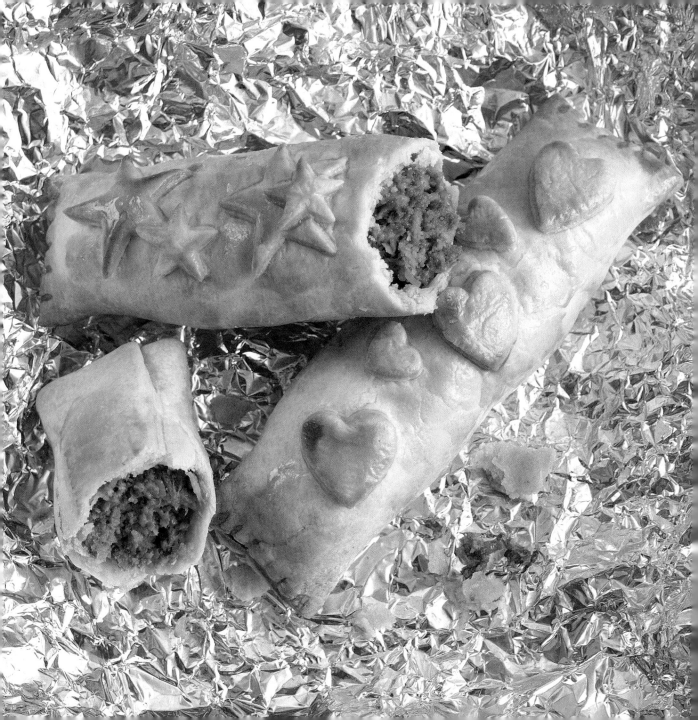

Beefy Hand Pies

Handheld pies make great picnic and party finger food, as they are ready-wrapped in pastry. To add a slight twist, I like to use beef, but ground pork would also be good.

Put the oil in a small frying pan, add the onion, and sauté for 5 minutes, or until soft. Stir in the thyme and set aside. Put the bread in a food processor and whiz to crumbs. Add the sautéed onion, beef, ketchup, and Parmesan, plus salt and pepper to taste, and whiz again to combine.

Preheat the oven to 400°F. Roll out the piecrust to 1/16 inch and trim into two rectangles about 7 × 5 inches. Halve the meat mixture and roll into two 7-inch sausages. Put one in the center of each rectangle of piecrust and brush the edges of the crust with egg. Roll the pastry over the meat to enclose it, and cut each roll into two pieces with a sharp knife (wipe the knife between each cut). Crimp the open ends of each pie with a fork to seal. Put the pies on a baking sheet, seam side down. Cut decorations, such as hearts or stars, from the leftover piecrust. Brush the pies with egg and attach the decorations, then brush the decorations with egg.

Bake the pies for 18 to 20 minutes, until the pastry is golden brown. Use a thin spatula to transfer the pies to a wire rack to cool. They are most delicious served warm, but can be served cold. They will keep in the fridge for up to 2 days.

🍳 Preparation 20 minutes
🕐 Cook 20 minutes
🍥 Makes 4 hand pies
❄ Suitable for freezing, unbaked, for up to 1 month. Thaw overnight in the fridge and bake as directed. Suitable for reheating at 215°F for about 15 minutes.

1 1/2 teaspoons olive oil
1/2 small red onion, chopped
1/4 teaspoon fresh thyme leaves
1 slice white bread, crusts removed
1/4 pound ground beef
1 tablespoon ketchup
2 tablespoons freshly grated Parmesan
salt and pepper, to season
one 7.5-ounce store-bought refrigerated piecrust
1 egg, beaten with a pinch of salt

TIP
Leftover piecrust can be used to make Mini Bacon and Egg Tarts (page 106).

Minty Lamb Koftas

🥘 Preparation 20 minutes
🕐 Cook 10 minutes
🍥 Makes 8 koftas
❄ Not suitable for freezing.
Leftovers will keep for up to
2 days in the fridge. Suitable for
reheating (skewers removed).
Reheat in a microwave for 20 to
30 seconds per kofta; otherwise
wrap meat in foil and bake at
350°F for 15 minutes.

1 small red onion, finely chopped
1 tablespoon olive oil
1 garlic clove, crushed
½ teaspoon ground cumin
½ pound ground lamb
⅓ cup fresh bread crumbs, from
   1 slice white bread, crusts
   removed
2 teaspoons chopped fresh mint
   leaves
1 teaspoon honey
1 egg yolk
salt and pepper, to season

You will also need 8 wooden
   skewers, soaked in warm
   water for 30 minutes

Children love to eat things on sticks, and sometimes I have called these "lamb pops" to increase the appeal. However, the koftas are also good stuffed into pitas or wraps (remove the skewers first) or even as slightly larger lamb burgers. Try them with my Minty Yogurt Dressing (page 38).

Sauté the onion in the oil for 5 to 6 minutes, or until soft. Add the garlic and cumin, and cook for an extra minute, then transfer to a bowl. Add the remaining ingredients, seasoning to taste with the salt and pepper, and mix thoroughly. For a finer texture, pulse everything in a food processor.

Divide the mixture into eighths and form into balls. Thread a skewer through each ball and use your hand firmly to form each ball into a sausage shape on the skewer. If possible, chill the koftas for 1 to 2 hours.

Preheat the broiler. Broil the koftas for 8 to 10 minutes, turning halfway, until cooked through. Let cool slightly before serving, and remove from the skewers for smaller children.

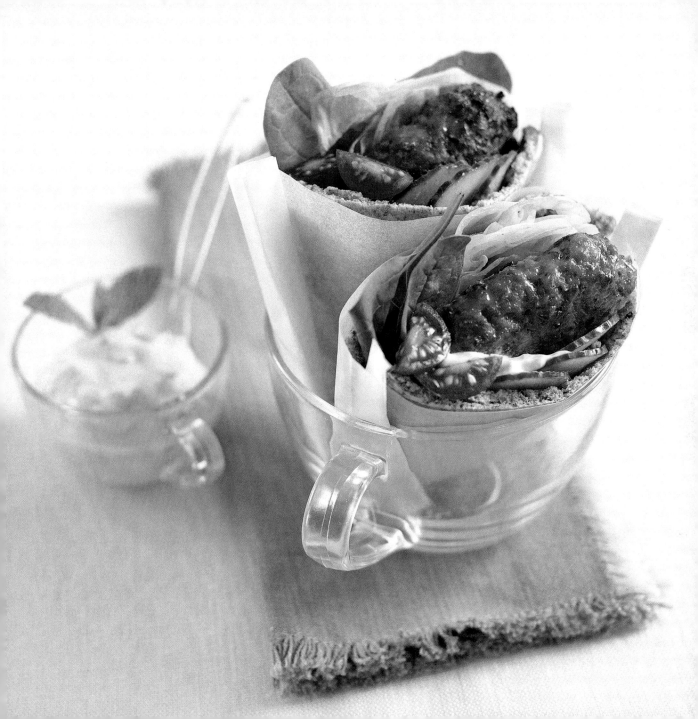

Simply Snacks

When children come home from day care or school, they are usually starving, so it's a good idea to have some healthy snacks ready on the table so that they don't just grab a bag of potato chips and a chocolate cookie. Simple things can make all the difference. Whole fruit in a bowl tends to go uneaten, but it will be much more appealing if you spend a few minutes cutting it up and arranging it on a plate, or threading bite-size pieces onto a straw.

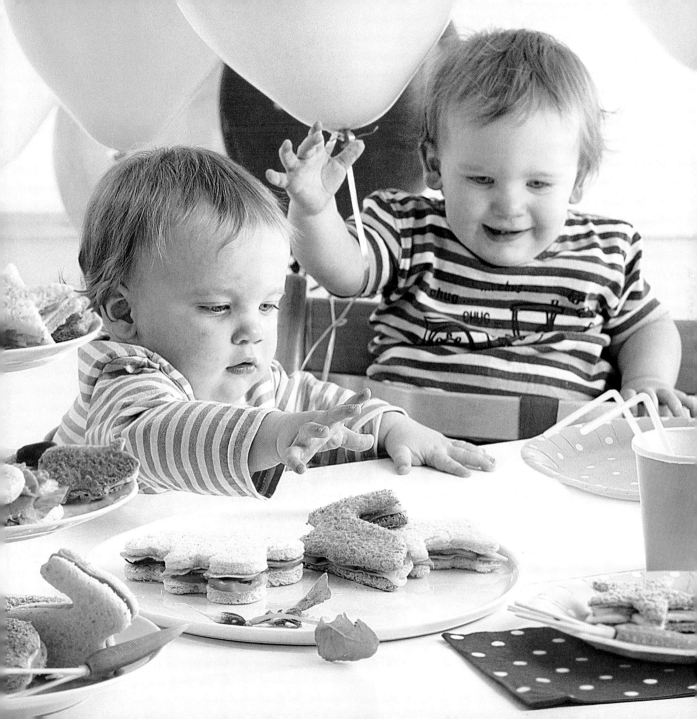

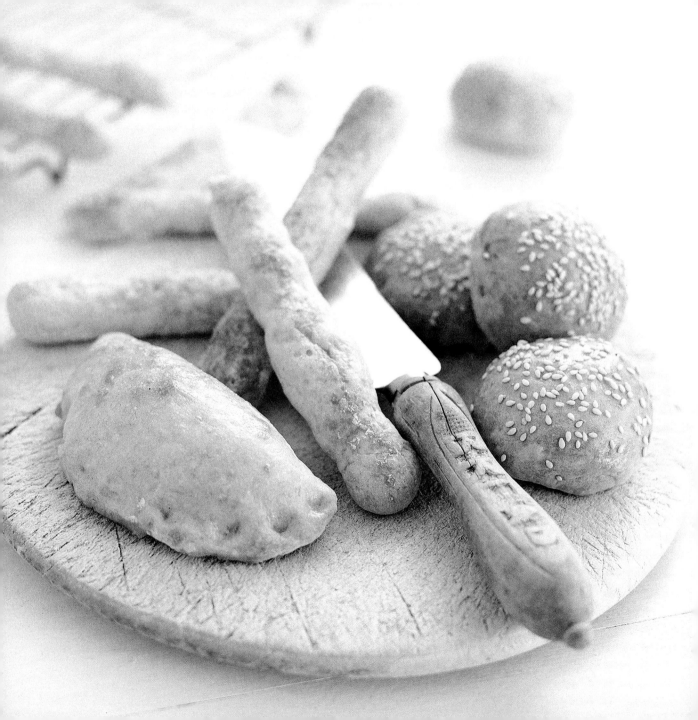

Basic Bread Dough— and Three Ways to Use It

Dissolve the yeast and sugar in a small bowl using ¼ cup of the water. Let stand for 5 minutes—it should start to turn frothy.

Mix the flour and salt in a large bowl, then add the yeast mixture, oil, and the remaining water. Mix to a soft dough, adding 1 to 2 teaspoons of extra water if the dough seems too dry.

Turn the dough onto a lightly floured surface and knead for around 10 minutes, until the dough feels smooth and springy. Put the dough in a large, lightly oiled bowl and cover with a clean, damp cloth. Leave to rise in a warm place for 45 minutes to 1 hour, until doubled in size.

Turn out the dough onto a floured surface and knead for 1 minute, then use for one of the three recipes that follow.

Preparation 20 minutes, plus rising

one ¼-ounce envelope active dry yeast
1 teaspoon sugar
⅔ cup water, 105° to 110°F
2 cups bread flour, or 1 cup bread flour and 1 cup whole wheat flour
¼ teaspoon salt (omit for children under 1 year)
1 tablespoon olive oil

Cheesy Breadsticks

Preheat the oven to 300°F.

Divide the dough into 20 equal pieces (about ½ ounce each) and keep covered with a clean, damp cloth. Take one piece and form it into a sausage shape, then roll out to a stick approximately 7 inches long and about the thickness of a little finger. Transfer to a lightly oiled baking sheet and cover with plastic wrap while you shape the other breadsticks. Space the breadsticks at least 1 inch apart on the baking sheet. Brush the breadsticks with the beaten egg and sprinkle with the cheese. Bake for 18 to 20 minutes for soft breadsticks or 30 to 35 minutes for crisp. Let cool on a wire rack. Soft breadsticks will keep in an airtight container for 1 day; crisp, for 5 days.

Preparation 45 minutes, plus rising
Cook 20 to 35 minutes
Makes 20 breadsticks
Suitable for children under 1
Suitable for freezing: The breadsticks can be frozen after baking.

1 recipe Basic Bread Dough
olive oil, for greasing
1 egg, beaten
⅓ cup freshly grated Parmesan

Baby Burger Buns

Preparation 30 minutes, plus rising
Cook 14 minutes
Makes 12 buns
Baked buns are suitable for freezing. Thaw for 1 hour at room temperature, then reheat for 10 minutes in an oven at 225°F. To freeze unbaked buns, see directions at right.

1 recipe Basic Bread Dough
olive oil, for greasing
1 egg, beaten
1 teaspoon sesame seeds

Preheat the oven to 400°F.

Divide the dough into 12 equal pieces (about 1 ounce each) and form into balls. Transfer to a lightly oiled baking sheet and cover with a clean, damp cloth. Let rise for 10 to 15 minutes, until doubled in size.

Brush the tops with a little of the egg and sprinkle with the sesame seeds. Bake for 12 to 14 minutes, until golden and the base of the rolls sound hollow when tapped. Let cool on a wire rack.

The bread dough can be frozen after being shaped into balls. Freeze on a plastic wrap–lined baking sheet. When firm, transfer to freezer bags. To thaw, put as many rolls as you want to bake on a lightly greased baking sheet, cover with plastic wrap, and leave in a warm place for 2 to 3 hours, until doubled in size. Brush with egg, sprinkle with sesame seeds, and bake as above.

Mini Pizzas

Preparation 30 minutes, plus rising
Cook 12 minutes
Makes 6 mini pizzas
Suitable for freezing (right). Not suitable for reheating.

1 recipe Basic Bread Dough
olive oil, for greasing
1 tablespoon tomato or marinara sauce per pizza
1/4 cup grated mozzarella per pizza
toppings of your choice (e.g., ham, sliced mushrooms, pepperoni, sliced bell peppers)

Preheat the oven to 400°F.

Divide the dough into 6 portions (approximately 2 ounces each). Roll out each portion to a circle about 5 inches in diameter and transfer to lightly oiled baking sheets. Spread with the tomato sauce and sprinkle with the cheese, then add any toppings. Bake for 10 to 12 minutes, until the cheese is bubbling and golden, and the crusts are crisp.

Suitable for freezing: The unbaked dough can be frozen after it is divided. Freeze on plastic wrap–lined baking sheets. When firm, transfer to freezer bags. Thaw on baking sheets, covered with plastic wrap, for 1 1/2 to 2 hours at room temperature, then roll out the pizza crusts and continue as above.

Mix 'n' Match Pasta Salad with Mild Mayo

Toddlers can be notoriously picky eaters, but getting them involved in the "preparation" of their meal can help to catch their attention and also make them feel as if they have some element of choice in the matter. Put the pasta on your toddler's plate and give a selection of add-in ingredients in small bowls so that he can pick out and add in what he likes. The mild mayo can be used as a dressing, but I often give it as a dip in a separate bowl, as it can make the salad a little slippery for small fingers.

Cook the pasta following the package instructions. Drain, rinse well with cold water, and drain in a colander for 5 minutes. Mix together the mayonnaise, water, and lemon juice and season to taste with salt and pepper. *(Continues on next page)*

Preparation 15 minutes
Cook 12 minutes
Makes 1 portion (easily doubled)

⅓ cup (or a large handful) large pasta shapes, such as bows (farfalle), spirals (fusilli), or corkscrews (cavatappi)
2 tablespoons mayonnaise
2 teaspoons water
¼ teaspoon fresh lemon juice
salt and pepper, to season

Protein Add-Ins
1 large slice ham, cut into strips
1 ounce thinly sliced roast beef, cut into small strips
1 ounce Cheddar, cut into matchsticks
1 ounce fresh mozzarella, cut into small cubes
1 ounce cooked chicken, torn into small strips
3 or 4 cold cooked Parmesan Chicken Strips (page 72)
Omelet Strips (page 118)
(Continued on next page)

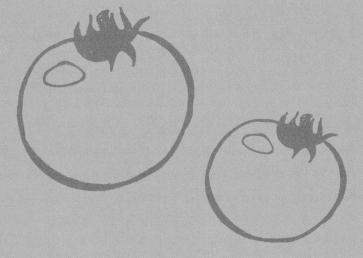

(Continued from page 117)

Salad Add-Ins

3 cherry or grape tomatoes, quartered

¼ small red, yellow, or orange bell pepper, cut into matchsticks

One 1-inch piece cucumber, peeled, seeded, and cut into thin half-moons

2 or 3 tablespoons drained canned corn

¼ apple, peeled, cored, and cut into thin slices

1 Grilled Vegetable Skewer (page 36), vegetables removed from skewer, or 1 ounce grilled vegetables from a delicatessen

½ medium carrot, cut into matchsticks

a small handful of lightly cooked broccoli florets

¼ cup bite-size green bean pieces, lightly cooked

4 pitted olives, quartered

a handful of bean sprouts

a small handful of shredded red cabbage

TIP

Cutting the vegetables into matchsticks encourages toddlers to bite and chew, but please make sure that your child is supervised at all times when eating.

Put the pasta on your child's plate and offer one or two protein add-ins and two or three salad add-ins (according to appetite), in separate bowls, to choose from. Once your child has assembled his salad, toss with the dressing or offer it as a dip. Leftover dressing and salad items will keep for 1 to 2 days in the fridge, tightly covered.

Omelet Strips

Whisk 1 egg with 1 tablespoon milk and season with salt and pepper to taste. Melt a pat of butter in an 8-inch frying pan and add the egg. Swirl around the pan to make a thin omelet. Cook for about 3 minutes, until set. Slide onto a plate and cut into strips.

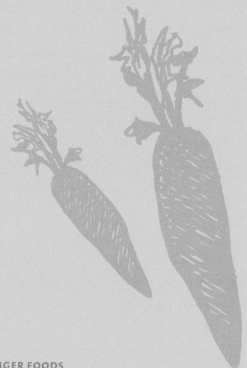

Lettuce Boats

Small lettuce leaves are custom made for yummy fillings. They are easy to pick up and a fun alternative to a sandwich or roll.

Each lettuce boat variation
Preparation 5 minutes
Makes 4 boats, 2 portions

Shrimp Cocktail

The shrimp filling is also delicious in a wrap, with a handful of shredded iceberg or romaine lettuce.

Put the mayonnaise, ketchup, sweet chili sauce, if using, and lemon juice for the sauce in a bowl, mix together, and season to taste with salt and pepper. Add the shrimp and toss to coat with the dressing. Divide the shrimp cocktail among the four lettuce leaves. Thread a toothpick through each of the lemon slices and secure one to each boat as a sail.

Chicken & Mango

You could substitute a quarter of a teaspoon of chopped fresh cilantro for the mint, if you like.

Mix together the yogurt, water, curry paste or powder, and honey in a bowl, and season to taste with salt and pepper. Add the chicken and mango and toss to coat with the dressing. Spoon the salad into the lettuce leaves and sprinkle with the chopped mint, if using.

Shrimp Cocktail
2 tablespoons mayonnaise
2 teaspoons ketchup
1/2 teaspoon sweet red chili sauce (optional)
1/4 teaspoon fresh lemon juice
salt and pepper, to season
1/4 pound cooked, peeled salad-size shrimp
4 small romaine lettuce leaves
4 toothpicks, to decorate
4 thin slices lemon, to decorate

Chicken & Mango
2 tablespoons Greek-style yogurt
1/2 teaspoon water
1/4 teaspoon korma or mild curry paste (such as Patak's), or a pinch of mild curry powder (or to taste)
1/4 teaspoon honey
salt and pepper, to season
2 ounces cooked chicken, diced (about 1/4 cup)
1/2 small ripe mango, pitted, peeled, and diced
4 small romaine lettuce leaves
2 small fresh mint leaves, chopped (optional)

Prosciutto and Taleggio Panini

Preparation 5 minutes
Cook 5 minutes
Makes 1 portion
Not suitable for freezing or reheating

1 slice prosciutto or Parma ham
1 hot dog bun, split down the side
2 ounces Taleggio, orange rind removed, thinly sliced
olive oil, for greasing

Hot dog buns are just right for baby panini, and the deliciously creamy Taleggio cheese in this filling (which I first ate on a mountainside in Italy) melts beautifully. You could use fontina or mozzarella instead.

Preheat a ridged grill pan, heavy-bottomed frying pan, or panini press. Lay the prosciutto on the base of the hot dog bun, folding it in to fit. Set the cheese on top of the prosciutto and sandwich with the top half of the bun, pressing down well.

Grease the pan with a little olive oil and set the filled bun, top side down, in the hot pan. Press down firmly with a spatula and cook for 2 minutes, until the top of the bun is crisp and golden. Carefully turn the bun over and cook for 2 to 3 minutes more, until the base of the bun is crisp and the cheese has melted.

Transfer to a plate and allow to cool slightly. Cut in half or into quarters to serve.

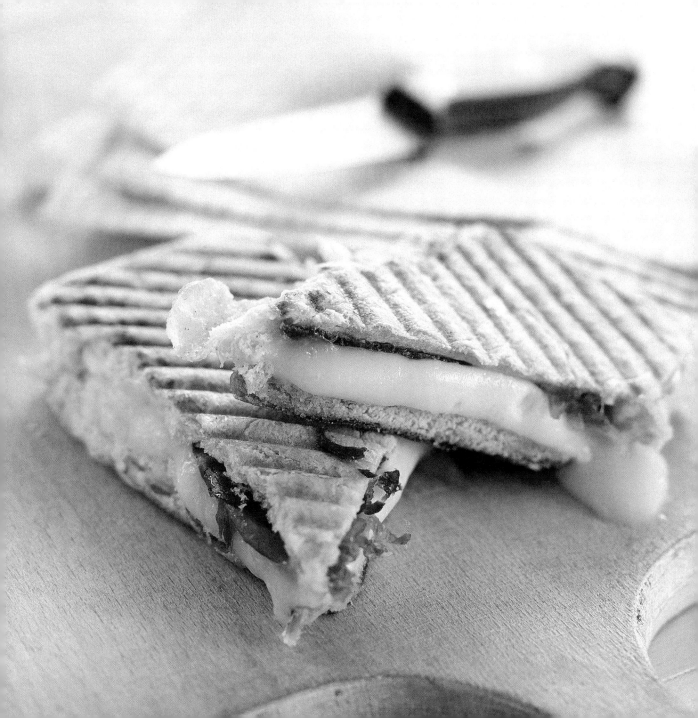

Tuna Muffin Melts

Preparation 5 minutes
Cook 5 minutes
Makes 2 to 4 portions (recipe easily halved)
Not suitable for freezing or reheating

one 6-ounce can tuna, drained
1 scallion, finely chopped
2 tablespoons Greek-style yogurt
2 tablespoons ketchup
1/4 teaspoon fresh lemon juice
2 drops Worcestershire sauce (optional)
salt and pepper, to season
2 English muffins, split in half
1/3 cup grated Cheddar

Halved and toasted English muffins are an ideal size for smaller children to pick up and eat. Don't be put off if the tuna filling makes more than you need—it keeps, covered, in the fridge for 2 to 3 days and makes a good sandwich or quesadilla filling. For a quesadilla, spread half of the tuna mix on a 7-inch flour tortilla, sprinkle with half the cheese, top with a second tortilla, and dry-fry or broil for around 2 minutes on each side, until crisp.

Preheat the broiler.

Put the tuna and scallion in a bowl and stir in the yogurt, ketchup, lemon juice, and Worcestershire sauce, if using. Season to taste with salt and pepper.

Lightly toast the muffins. Pile the tuna mix on the cut sides. Sprinkle with the cheese and broil for 1 to 2 minutes, until the cheese has melted. Let cool slightly, then serve cut in half or into quarters.

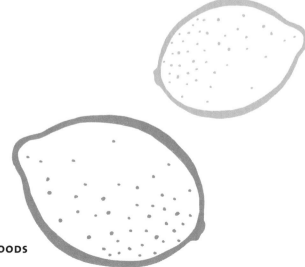

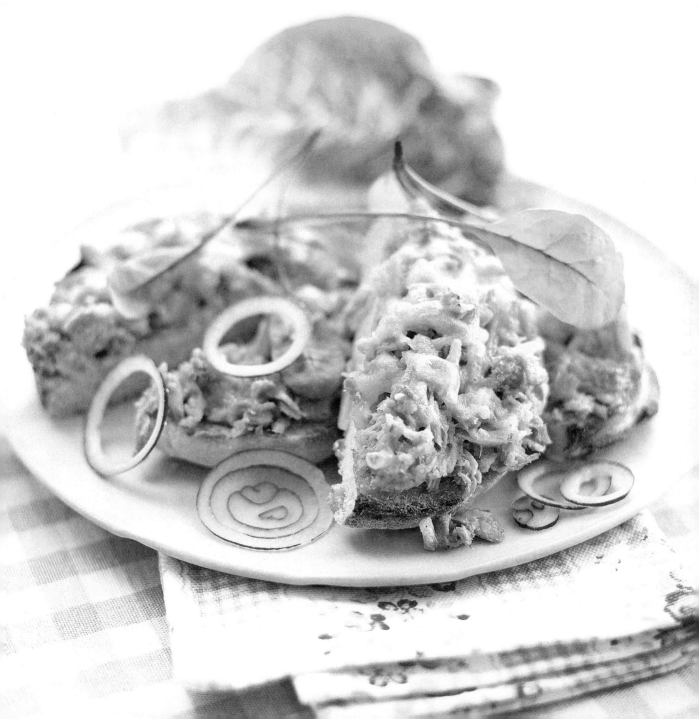

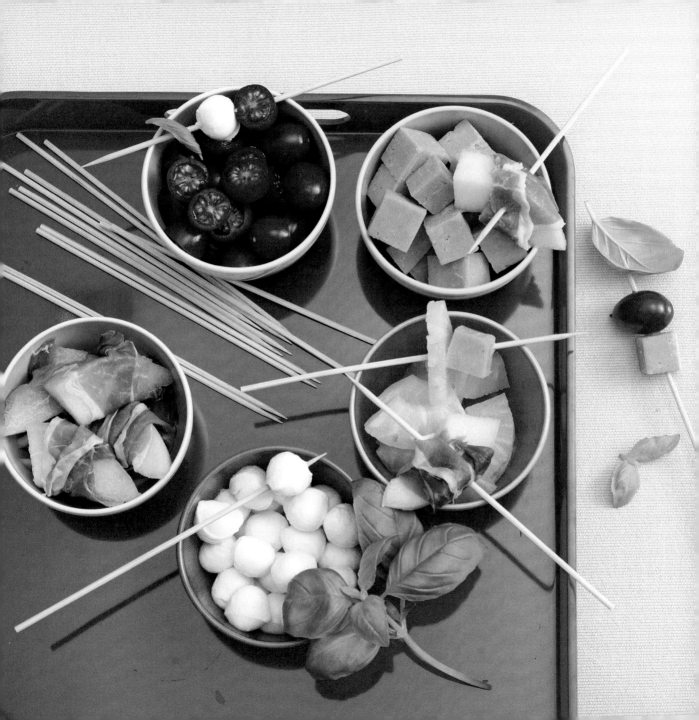

Salad Lollipops

Salad lollipops make a nice change from a sandwich in a lunch box. It's best to remove the skewers for younger children. Or use thin drinking straws instead to secure the ingredients.

Cheese & Pineapple

For a fun party presentation, spear the skewers into the skin of a halved grapefruit to look like a hedgehog.

Thread a cube of cheese and a halved cube of pineapple onto each skewer. Top with a halved cherry or grape tomato, if using.

Tomato & Mozzarella

If making these for a lunch box, it is best to scrape the seeds out of the halved tomatoes to prevent the lollipops from becoming soggy, or use whole tomatoes.

Season the mozzarella with salt and pepper to taste. Thread half of a cherry or grape tomato onto a skewer, followed by a piece of mozzarella and another tomato half. Finish with a basil leaf, if using. This is good served with my Balsamic Dip (page 126).

Each salad lollipop variation
- Preparation 10 minutes
- Makes 8 lollipops, 2 portions
- Not suitable for freezing

Cheese & Pineapple
2 ounces mild Cheddar, cut into eight 1/2-inch cubes
4 cubes canned pineapple, drained and cut in half
4 cherry or grape tomatoes, halved (optional)

You will also need 8 skewers

Tomato & Mozzarella
4 small mozzarella balls (bocconcini), halved, or 2 ounces fresh mozzarella, cut into eight 1/2-inch cubes
salt and pepper, to season
8 cherry or grape tomatoes, halved
8 small fresh basil leaves (optional)
Balsamic Dip (page 126), to serve (optional)

You will also need 8 skewers

Prosciutto & Melon
¼ Galia melon or cantaloupe,
    seeded and rind removed
4 slices prosciutto or Parma ham,
    or 4 wafer-thin slices ham
pepper, to season
Balsamic Dip, to serve (optional)

You will also need 8 toothpicks

Balsamic Dip
🖐 Preparation 5 minutes
🍽 Makes 2 portions

1 tablespoon olive oil
1 teaspoon balsamic vinegar
½ teaspoon honey (or to taste)
salt and pepper, to season

Prosciutto & Melon

Cut 8 cubes (each about ½ inch) from the melon. Cut the prosciutto in half lengthwise and slightly fold in the long edges of each piece to give neat strips. Wrap 1 strip of prosciutto around a melon cube and thread onto a toothpick. Repeat with the remaining prosciutto and melon. Season to taste with pepper. This is nice served with my Balsamic Dip, below.

Balsamic Dip

Whisk together the oil, vinegar, and honey and season to taste with salt and pepper. Serve in small bowls.

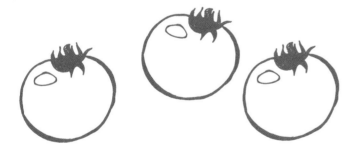
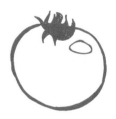
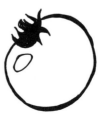

Ham and Cheese Quesadilla

Grilled ham and cheese sandwiches are perennially popular—using a flour tortilla makes a thin, crisp sandwich that will appeal to all ages.

Preheat a heavy frying pan (no need to grease) or preheat the broiler. Cut the tortilla in half. Sprinkle half of the cheese on one piece of the tortilla, then set the ham on top. Sprinkle with the remaining cheese and top with the second piece of tortilla. Press down slightly. Cook in the frying pan for 1½ to 2 minutes, until the base is brown and crisp. Flip the tortilla over using a spatula and cook for 1½ to 2 minutes more, until the cheese has melted. If you prefer, you can also broil the quesadilla for 1½ to 2 minutes on each side.

   Transfer to a plate and let cool slightly before cutting into triangles or strips to serve.

Preparation 5 minutes
Cook 4 minutes
Makes 1 portion (recipe easily doubled)
Not suitable for freezing or reheating

one 7-inch flour tortilla
¼ cup grated Cheddar
1 or 2 thin slices ham

Chicken Fajitas with Mild Salsa

🍽 Preparation 20 minutes
🕐 Cook 7 minutes
🍲 Makes 2 portions
❄ Not suitable for freezing

For the Mild Salsa
1 large tomato, peeled, seeded, and diced
1 scallion, thinly sliced
2 teaspoons chopped fresh cilantro (or to taste)
1 teaspoon fresh lime juice
salt and pepper, to season

2 teaspoons ketchup
1 teaspoon balsamic vinegar
1 teaspoon water
1/2 teaspoon brown sugar
a pinch of dried oregano
2 drops Tabasco sauce (optional)
1 teaspoon canola oil
1 boneless, skinless chicken breast, sliced into thin strips (about 5 ounces)
1 medium red onion, thinly sliced
1/4 small red bell pepper, seeded and thinly sliced
1/4 small yellow bell pepper, seeded and thinly sliced
two 7-inch flour tortillas
2 tablespoons Mild Salsa
1/4 cup sour cream
1 tablespoon guacamole (optional)

A lot of Mexican food is street food—it has evolved to be eaten with the hands and makes ideal finger food. If your child doesn't like bell peppers, just substitute a little extra chicken. Any leftover filling will keep, covered, in the fridge for up to 2 days. Reheat for 1 minute in a microwave or in the oven, wrapped in foil, for 10 minutes at 400°F.

To make the salsa, mix all of the ingredients together in a small bowl, seasoning to taste with salt and pepper. Cover and chill until needed—it will keep for up to 2 days in the fridge. Alternatively, use a mild store-bought salsa.

For the fajita filling, mix together the ketchup, balsamic vinegar, water, sugar, oregano, and Tabasco, if using, in a small bowl and set aside.

Heat the oil in a large pan or wok and stir-fry the chicken for 2 minutes. Add the vegetables and stir-fry for 3 to 4 minutes more, until the chicken has cooked through and the vegetables have softened slightly. Add the ketchup mixture and cook, stirring, for 1 minute more. Remove from the heat.

Warm the tortillas for 10 to 15 seconds in a microwave, or for 1 minute on each side in a dry frying pan. Spoon the fajita filling down the center of each tortilla and top with the salsa, sour cream, and guacamole, if using. Roll up and serve immediately.

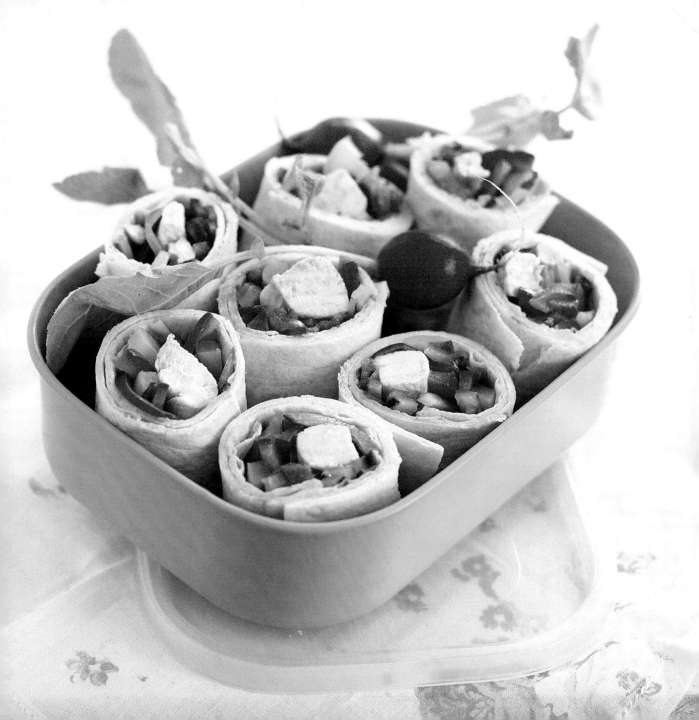

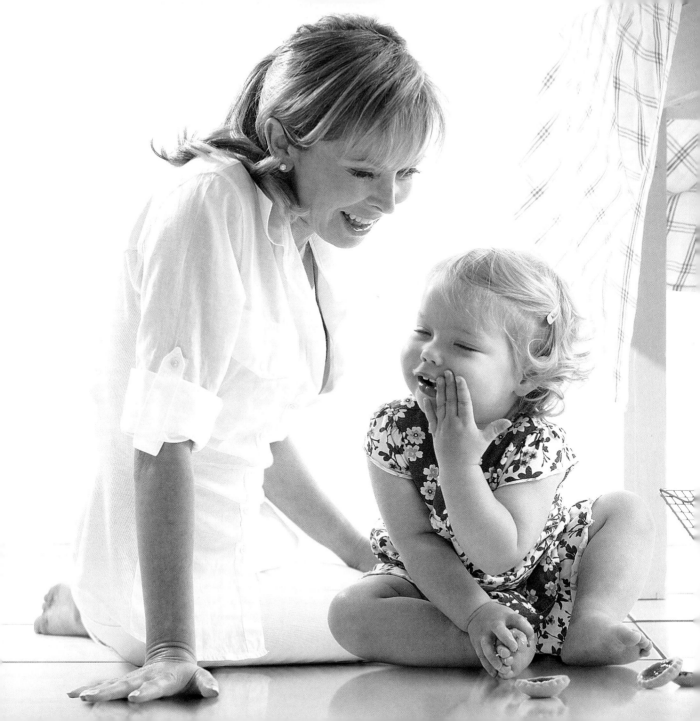

Sweet Treats

Well, of course, the best sweet finger food has to be fresh fruit—whether it's peeled clementines, pineapple chunks or strawberries threaded onto a skewer, or wedges of peeled mango or melon. If your child isn't keen on fresh fruit, you can always puree and freeze it in ice pop molds. I do think, though, that children need treats occasionally—so as well as wholesome recipes like Zucchini, Orange, and Spice Muffins and Oat and Raisin Cookies, I have included recipes for brownies and Mini Jam Tarts. After all, you are only a child once!

Apricot and White Chocolate Cereal Bars

⏱ Preparation 10 minutes, plus chilling
🕐 Cook 2 minutes
🍽 Makes 16 bars
❄ Not suitable for freezing

1³/₄ cups quick-cooking oats
1²/₃ cups Rice Krispies
¹/₃ cup chopped dried apricots (about 6 apricots)
¹/₂ cup chopped pecans (optional)
7 tablespoons butter
¹/₃ cup golden syrup (such as Lyle's)
heaping ¹/₃ cup white chocolate chips, or 2¹/₂ ounces white chocolate, chopped
a pinch of salt

These chewy bars taste delicious and don't need any baking. Children enjoy making them, as they are very quick and easy to prepare.

Combine the oats, Rice Krispies, apricots, and pecans, if using, in a mixing bowl. Put the butter, golden syrup, white chocolate, and salt in a large saucepan and heat gently, stirring occasionally, until melted together. Stir the oat and Rice Krispies mixture into the melted chocolate mixture until well coated.

Press the mixture into a shallow 11 × 7-inch pan lined with parchment paper, using a potato masher. Place in the fridge for about 2 hours to set, then cut into bars. Store in an airtight container in the fridge.

Carrot, Coconut, and Pineapple Muffins

Carrot and pineapple together make deliciously moist muffins. As they have a high fruit content, these muffins are best stored in the freezer.

Preheat the oven to 350°F. Line two mini muffin pans with paper cases (or line 8 holes of a standard muffin pan).

Whisk together the flour, baking powder, baking soda, cinnamon, and salt in a large bowl. In a separate bowl, mix together the melted butter, vanilla, egg, carrot, pineapple and juice, coconut, and brown sugar. Mix the wet ingredients into the dry ones, along with the raisins.

Spoon the mixture into the paper cases (three-quarters full) and bake for 12 to 14 minutes (for mini muffins) or 20 minutes (for regular-size muffins), until risen and firm to the touch. Let cool on a wire rack.

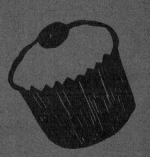

🥮 Preparation 15 minutes
🕐 Cook 14 minutes (mini)/ 20 minutes (regular)
🧁 Makes 24 mini or 8 regular muffins
❄ Suitable for freezing: Freeze baked muffins in a resealable container or freezer bag. Thaw at room temperature for 30 to 45 minutes (mini) or 2 hours (regular).

1¹⁄₃ cups whole wheat flour, or
   ²⁄₃ cup whole wheat flour and
   ²⁄₃ cup all-purpose flour
1 teaspoon baking powder
¹⁄₂ teaspoon baking soda
¹⁄₂ teaspoon ground cinnamon
¹⁄₄ teaspoon salt
6 tablespoons (³⁄₄ stick) butter, melted
1 teaspoon vanilla extract
1 egg
1 medium carrot, finely grated
¹⁄₄ cup drained canned crushed pineapple (reserve juice)
1 tablespoon pineapple juice
¹⁄₂ cup unsweetened shredded coconut (see tip on page 67)
¹⁄₂ cup (packed) plus 1 tablespoon light brown sugar
¹⁄₃ cup raisins (chopped for smaller children)

Yogurt, Orange, and Lemon Mini Cupcakes

🍲 Preparation 15 minutes
🕐 Cook 20 minutes
🍪 Makes 18 mini cupcakes
☺ Suitable for children under 1
❄ Suitable for freezing:
Un-iced cupcakes can be frozen
in a resealable container or
freezer bag.

4 tablespoons (½ stick) butter,
   softened
½ cup superfine sugar
1 egg, at room temperature
finely grated zest of ½ small
   lemon
finely grated zest of ½ lime
½ teaspoon finely grated
   orange zest
1 heaping cup self-rising flour
3 tablespoons whole milk plain
   yogurt

For the icing
2 cups confectioners' sugar
1 tablespoon fresh orange juice
1 tablespoon fresh lime juice

These cute cupcakes are manageable mini mouthfuls for little
ones. Adding some yogurt and citrus fruit keeps them lovely
and moist and gives them a deliciously refreshing flavor. They
would be great for birthday parties.

Preheat the oven to 350°F and line two mini muffin pans with
18 paper cases.

   Cream the butter and sugar until pale and fluffy. Gradually
add the egg, beating well between additions. Stir in the zests.
Sift in the flour and fold in well. Stir in the yogurt. Divide the
mixture among the mini muffin cups. Bake for 18 to 20 minutes,
until risen, lightly golden brown, and firm to the touch. Let cool
in the pan for 5 minutes, then transfer to a wire rack and let
cool completely.

   Meanwhile, to make the icing, sift the confectioners' sugar
into a bowl. Make a well in the middle, stir in the juices, and
beat well. Spoon the icing onto the cooled cupcakes and allow
to set for up to 30 minutes. Store in an airtight container for
up to 5 days.

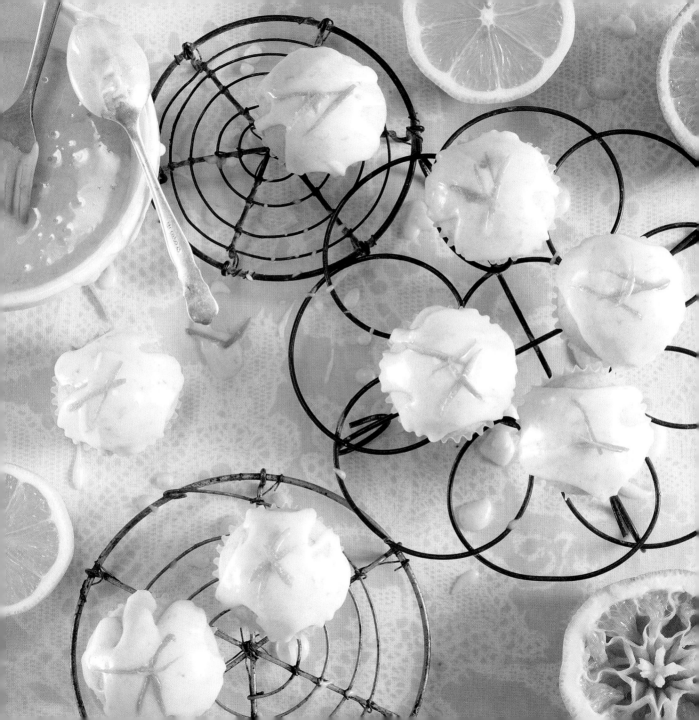

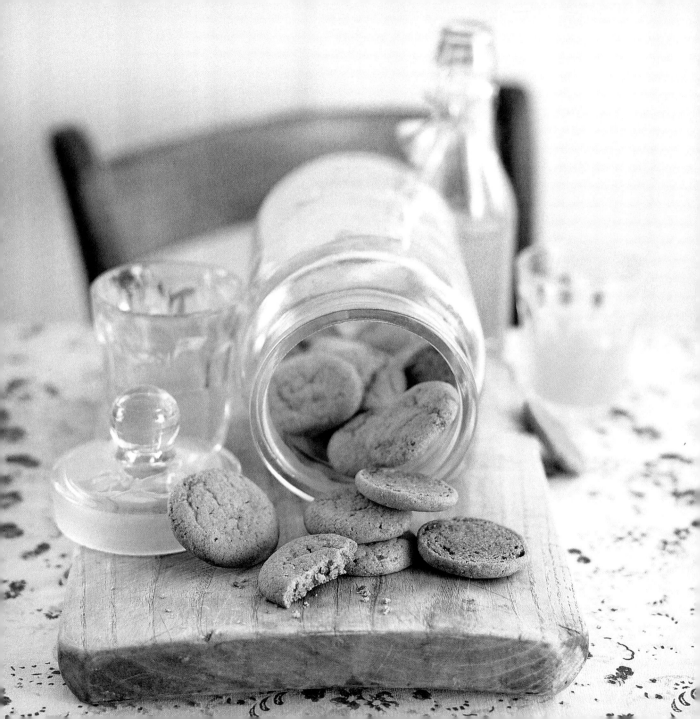

Gingersnaps

Children are very fond of crisp ginger cookies, and these little gingersnaps fit the bill perfectly. Dipping the teaspoon in water when scooping the dough will help to give you beautifully round cookies. These are extremely yummy and so easy to prepare.

Preheat the oven to 300°F.

Beat the butter, brown sugar, egg yolk, and syrup together in a large bowl until fluffy and slightly paler in color. Whisk together the dry ingredients, then add to the butter mixture and mix to form a soft dough.

Dip a round measuring teaspoon in a glass of water and scoop up a slightly rounded teaspoon of the dough. Drop it onto a cookie sheet lined with parchment paper. Continue dipping the teaspoon and scooping the remaining dough, leaving about 2 inches between each mound of dough, as the cookies will spread. You may need to bake the cookies in batches.

Bake the cookies for 14 to 16 minutes, until light brown around the edges. Remove from the oven and let cool for 5 minutes, then use a thin spatula to transfer the cookies to a wire rack. The cookies will continue to crisp up as they cool.

Store in an airtight container.

Preparation 20 minutes
Cook 16 minutes
Makes about 28 gingersnaps
Suitable for freezing: The baked and cooled cookies can be frozen for up to 1 month.

4 tablespoons (½ stick) butter, softened
½ cup (packed) plus 1 tablespoon light brown sugar
1 egg yolk
2 tablespoons golden syrup (such as Lyle's)
1 cup all-purpose flour
2 teaspoons ground ginger
¼ teaspoon baking soda
a pinch of salt (optional)

TIP
Bake for 2 to 3 minutes less for a chewier cookie.

Zucchini, Orange, and Spice Muffins

🍲 Preparation 15 minutes
🕐 Cook 14 minutes (mini)/
25 minutes (regular)
🍥 Makes 24 mini or 12 regular
muffins
☺ Suitable for children under 1
❄ Suitable for freezing. Thaw
for 1 hour at room temperature.

1 cup plus 2 tablespoons whole
    wheat flour
1/2 teaspoon baking powder
1/2 teaspoon baking soda
3/4 teaspoon pumpkin pie spice
a pinch of salt
juice and finely grated zest of
    1 medium orange
3 tablespoons butter, melted
1 egg
1/4 cup (packed) plus 1 tablespoon
    light brown sugar
1 small zucchini, finely grated
1/3 cup raisins, chopped (can
    leave whole for older children)

I have chopped the raisins for the mini muffins, making them easier for small children to eat, but you can leave them whole if baking regular-size muffins.

Preheat the oven to 350°F. Line two mini muffin pans with 24 paper cases, or line a 12-hole pan for regular muffins.

In a large bowl, whisk together the flour, baking powder, baking soda, pumpkin pie spice, and salt (omit salt for under-1-year-olds). Set aside.

Measure the orange juice—you need 7 tablespoons. If it is less, make up the quantity with milk or juice from a carton. Whisk the juice, zest, butter, egg, and brown sugar together until well combined, then stir into the flour mixture, followed by the zucchini and raisins. Spoon into the muffin cases (fill almost to the top). Bake for 12 to 14 minutes (increase the baking time to 22 to 25 minutes for regular-size muffins), until firm to the touch. Let cool on a wire rack. Store in an airtight container for up to 3 days.

Cinnamon Rolls

As they bake, these rolls fill the house with the delicious scent of cinnamon—perfect at breakfast or after school. Their small size makes them particularly child-friendly.

Beat the butter, brown sugar, and cinnamon until well combined. Roll out the dough into a rectangle approximately 14 × 7 inches and transfer to a lightly floured board or work surface. Spread the cinnamon butter over the surface of the dough, leaving a ½-inch border on one of the long edges. Roll up the dough into a long cylinder, starting from the long edge with the cinnamon butter and pressing gently to seal the dough roll.

Preheat the oven to 350°F.

Cut the cylinder into 12 slices with a sharp knife that has been lightly dusted with flour. Arrange, cut side up, on a lightly oiled baking sheet, in a rectangle of four rolls across and three rolls down, ½ inch apart, with the seams facing inward. Cover with a clean, damp cloth and let rise for 15 to 20 minutes, until puffy and doubled in size (the rolls should touch each other lightly).

Brush the tops and sides of the rolls with a little of the beaten egg. Bake for 18 to 20 minutes, until the rolls are golden and the bases sound hollow when tapped. Let cool slightly on the baking sheet.

Put the confectioners' sugar in a small bowl and add the water, a few drops at a time, until you have a thick but pourable icing. Drizzle over the rolls, then break them into individual portions. The rolls are nicest served warm. Leftover rolls can be stored for 1 day in an airtight container—gently reheat for 5 minutes in an oven preheated to 210°F.

⊙ Preparation 35 minutes, plus rising
🕐 Cook 20 minutes
◉ Makes 12 small rolls
❄ Suitable for freezing: Can be frozen un-iced after baking. Reheat as directed.

2 tablespoons butter, softened
2 tablespoons light brown sugar
½ teaspoon ground cinnamon
1 recipe Basic Bread Dough (page 115), replacing the olive oil with 1 tablespoon melted butter, risen once
1 egg, beaten

For the icing
¼ cup confectioners' sugar
approximately 1 teaspoon water

Super Strawberry Yogurt Ripple Cones

🍴 Preparation 15 minutes, plus churning and freezing
🍥 Makes 6 to 8 portions
☺ Suitable for children under 1

8 ounces strawberries, hulled and halved
½ teaspoon fresh lemon juice
¼ cup superfine sugar
1¾ cups whole milk plain yogurt
½ cup good-quality strawberry jam (such as Bonne Maman)
1 cup heavy cream
ice-cream cones, to serve

Ice-cream cones are irresistible to all age groups—and making ice cream with yogurt is extremely easy, as you can just mix everything together. I love strawberry ice cream and strawberry sorbet—and this ripple ice cream gives me a little of each!

Put the strawberries, lemon juice, and half of the sugar in a blender, and whiz to a puree. Taste the puree and add more of the sugar to sweeten, if necessary. You can strain the puree to remove the seeds, if you like. You should have just under 1 cup of puree.

Put the yogurt in a large bowl and stir in the jam plus half of the puree. Whip the cream to soft peaks in a separate bowl, then fold the cream into the yogurt mixture. Pour this ice cream base into an ice cream maker and churn according to the manufacturer's instructions.

Transfer the frozen ice cream to a resealable container. Spoon on the remaining strawberry puree, and ripple through the ice cream with a knife or metal skewer. Cover and store in the freezer for up to 1 month.

To serve, scoop balls of the ice cream into cones. If the ice cream is too hard to scoop, let it soften slightly at room temperature for 5 to 10 minutes.

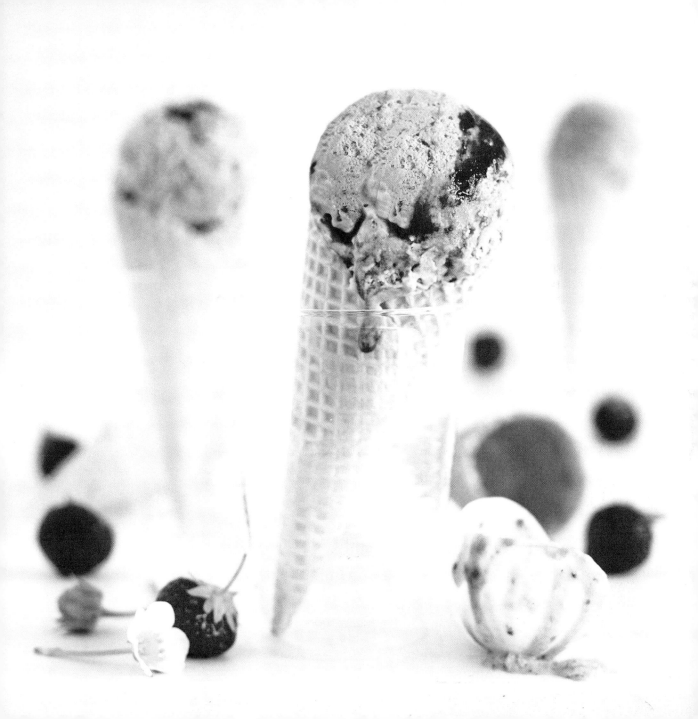

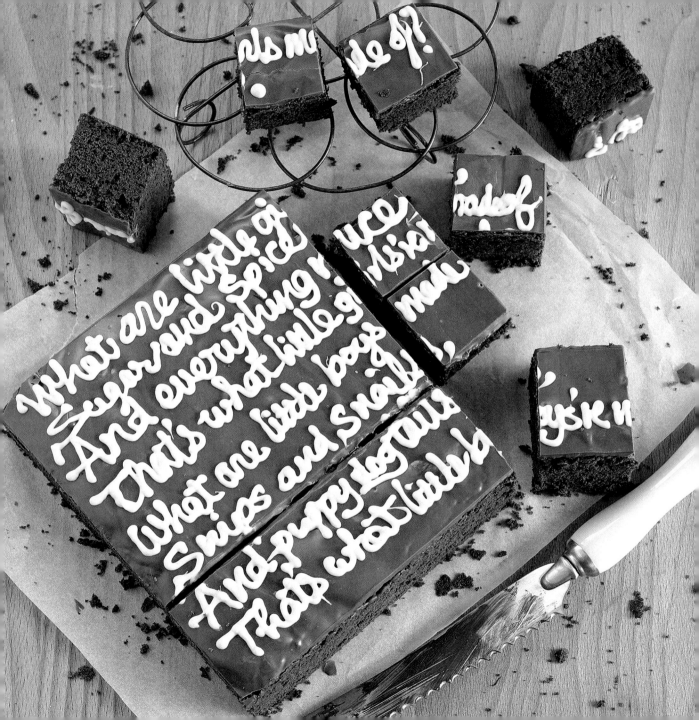

Brownie Bites

Preheat the oven to 350°F. Line the base and sides of a 13 × 9-inch baking pan with parchment paper.

Put the bittersweet chocolate, butter, and sugar in a heatproof bowl, and melt over a saucepan of simmering water (don't let the bottom of the bowl touch the water). Alternatively, melt in a microwave in 15-second bursts, stirring between bursts. Set aside to cool.

Whisk together the eggs and vanilla until just combined, and stir into the cooled chocolate. Sift the flour, cocoa, baking powder, and salt on top and mix in. Pour the batter into the prepared pan and bake for 25 to 30 minutes, until a skewer inserted into the center comes out with damp crumbs clinging to it (but not uncooked brownie batter)—try not to overbake. Remove from the oven and let cool in the pan.

When the brownie base is cold, make the topping. Put the milk chocolate, butter, and cream in a heatproof bowl and carefully melt (as above). Stir until smooth, then spread over the top of the brownie. Put the white chocolate in a separate bowl and carefully melt (as above). Spoon into the corner of a plastic bag, snip off the corner, and drizzle the white chocolate over the chocolate topping. Leave in a cool place (but not the fridge) until the topping is fully set.

Lift the brownie out of its pan using the parchment paper. Put on a cutting board and cut into 16 bars or 20 squares. Store in an airtight container in a cool place for up to 5 days.

Topping Variation

Melt ¾ cup milk chocolate chips and spread this over the top of the brownie. When it's set, pipe on words using the melted white chocolate or white writing icing.

🍮 Preparation 30 minutes
🕐 Cook 30 minutes
🍪 Makes 16 small bars or 20 small squares
❄ Suitable for freezing: Lift the cooled, uncut (un-iced) brownie from the pan and wrap in a double layer of plastic wrap followed by a single layer of foil. Thaw for 2 to 3 hours at room temperature before topping and cutting.

heaping 1 cup bittersweet
    chocolate chips, or 7 ounces
    bittersweet chocolate, chopped
2 sticks butter, cut into cubes
1¼ cups superfine sugar
3 eggs
1 teaspoon vanilla extract
1 cup all-purpose flour
2 tablespoons unsweetened
    cocoa powder
1 teaspoon baking powder
¼ teaspoon salt

For the topping
½ cup milk or bittersweet
    chocolate chips, or 4 ounces
    chocolate, chopped
1 tablespoon butter
2 tablespoons heavy cream
¼ cup white chocolate chips, or
    2 ounces white chocolate,
    chopped

Date and Honey
Cereal Bars

🍲 Preparation 35 minutes
🕐 Cook 20 minutes
🍥 Makes 16 squares
❄ Suitable for freezing: Wrap individually in plastic wrap or freeze in a resealable container or freezer bag. Thaw at room temperature.

3/4 cup chopped pitted dates
1 stick plus 2 tablespoons butter
heaping 1/3 cup sugar
1 tablespoon honey
1/2 teaspoon vanilla extract
1 tablespoon sesame seeds
2 1/2 cups quick-cooking oats
a pinch of salt
1/2 cup golden raisins
1/4 cup semisweet chocolate
   chips

A tasty snack to give your child long-lasting energy.

Preheat the oven to 350°F and line an 8-inch square pan with parchment paper. Put the dates in a small bowl and cover with boiling water. Let soften for 5 minutes.

Drain the dates and squeeze out any excess water. Put the butter, sugar, honey, and dates into a saucepan. Heat gently, stirring, until the butter melts and the dates become mushy, then remove from the heat. (If you like, you can pulse the mixture in a food processor or with a hand blender for a smoother texture.) Stir in the remaining ingredients except for the chocolate chips. Allow the mixture to cool a little, then stir in the chocolate chips (they will melt if you stir them in too soon).

Spoon the mixture into the prepared pan and press into an even layer. Bake for 20 minutes, then let stand for 10 minutes before cutting into 16 squares. Allow the squares to cool completely before removing from the pan. Store in an airtight container.

Oat and Raisin Cookies

These cookies not only are delicious but also have a dose of whole grains, with the whole wheat flour and rolled oats, which help to keep up energy levels.

Preheat the oven to 350°F.

Beat together the butter, brown sugar, and vanilla. Add all the dry ingredients and mix together. Form into balls using 1 tablespoon of the mixture and arrange spaced apart on two baking sheets lined with parchment paper.

Bake for about 12 minutes, until golden. Allow to firm up a little before transferring to a wire rack to cool completely.

🍲 Preparation 20 minutes
🕐 Cook 12 minutes
🍮 Makes 10 cookies
❄ Suitable for freezing

4 tablespoons (½ stick) butter, softened
¼ cup (packed) light brown sugar
½ teaspoon vanilla extract
¼ cup whole wheat flour
⅓ cup quick-cooking oats
¼ teaspoon ground cinnamon or pumpkin pie spice
¼ teaspoon salt
a pinch of baking soda
3 tablespoons raisins

Cottage Cheese Dip for Fruit

Cottage cheese is a great source of protein, but some children dislike the texture. However, you can blend the cheese until it is smooth to make a tasty dip for chunks of fruit. Add a swirl of fruit puree for a splash of color.

Blend the cottage cheese, milk, and honey together until smooth. Cover and chill the dip until ready to serve (it will keep in the fridge for 3 to 4 days).

To serve, spoon 2 to 3 tablespoons of the dip into small dishes, top with a teaspoon of fruit puree, and swirl with a toothpick. Serve with chunks of your child's favorite fruits, for dipping.

🍲 Preparation 5 minutes
🍮 Makes 4 to 6 portions
❄ Not suitable for freezing

1 cup cottage cheese (not fat-free)
2 tablespoons milk
1 teaspoon honey
4 to 6 teaspoons fruit jam, to serve
fruit chunks (e.g., apple slices, halved strawberries, pineapple cubes), to serve

Handheld Apple Pies

🍲 Preparation 30 minutes,
plus cooling
🕐 Cook 15 minutes
🍽 Makes 6 pies
❄ Suitable for freezing: Put the
unbaked pies on a baking sheet
lined with plastic wrap. Cover with
more plastic wrap and freeze for 3 to
4 hours, until solid, then transfer to
a resealable container. Bake directly
from frozen on a well-greased
baking sheet in an oven preheated
to 350°F. Brush the tops with melted
butter, bake for 20 minutes, then
increase the heat to 400°F and
bake for 5 to 8 minutes more, until
golden. Not suitable for reheating:
best eaten freshly baked, so extras
should be frozen unbaked, and
baked from frozen.

2 large apples, peeled and cored
   (I use Pink Lady)
2 tablespoons light brown sugar
1/4 teaspoon ground cinnamon
4 tablespoons (1/2 stick) butter,
   melted
6 large sheets filo pastry
1 teaspoon confectioners' sugar,
   to serve

TIP
I like to grate the apple, so it is
easier for small children to eat.

I have to admit it—these are inspired by the handheld apple
pies sold in a fast-food restaurant. But I have replaced the
heavy pastry with light, crispy filo pastry and filled them with
cinnamon-scented apple that isn't at all "gloopy." Filo can dry
out quickly, so keep the sheets covered with a damp tea towel.

Grate the apples into a microwavable bowl, add the brown sugar
and cinnamon, and toss to mix. Cover with plastic wrap, punch
a steam hole, and microwave for 3 to 4 minutes, until the apples
are softening but not mushy. Alternatively, simmer the apples
in a small saucepan for 4 to 5 minutes. Uncover and let stand
until cool, about 30 minutes.

Preheat the oven to 400°F. Grease a baking sheet with a little
of the melted butter.

Lay one filo sheet on a flat work surface and brush generously
with the melted butter. Fold in half (short end to short end) and
brush again with butter. Put a rounded tablespoonful of the
apple filling at one of the short ends of the folded filo and spread
out slightly, leaving a 3/4-inch border on either side. Fold in the
two long sides (partially covering the filling at the bottom) and
brush the folded-in margins with butter. Roll up from the filled
end to make a cylinder. Set the pie, seam side down, on the
prepared baking sheet and cover with a lightly dampened towel
or paper towels. Repeat with the remaining filo, butter, and
apple.

Brush the tops and sides of the pies with butter and bake
for 10 to 15 minutes, until golden. Allow to cool for around
30 minutes, then dust with the confectioners' sugar. The filling
can remain very hot, so I prefer to cut the pies in half to serve.

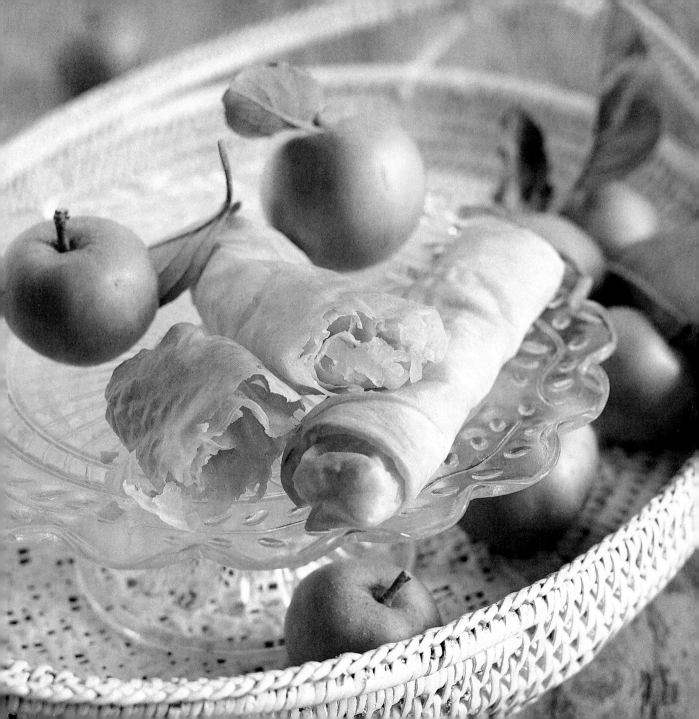

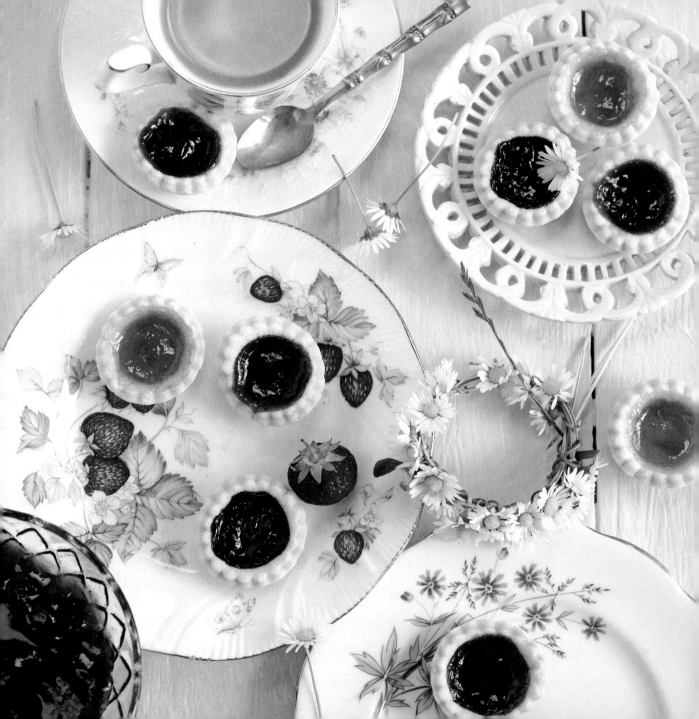

Mini Jam Tarts

Jewel-bright jam tarts are a yummy and easy-to-eat after-school treat, but can also be packed into lunch boxes. You can buy some very good sugar-free jams.

Preheat the oven to 350°F.

Unroll the piecrusts onto a lightly floured surface and use a 2-inch round cookie cutter to cut out 24 pastry circles. Gently push the pastry circles into the cups of mini muffin pans.

Drop half a teaspoonful of jam into the center of each pastry shell. Bake the tarts for 18 to 20 minutes, until the pastry is golden. Let cool for 5 minutes in the pan, then transfer to a wire rack to cool further. If eating warm, check the temperature of the tarts before serving, as the jam can get very hot. Store cooled tarts in an airtight container for 2 to 3 days.

Preparation 15 minutes
Cook 20 minutes
Makes 24 tarts
Suitable for freezing: Put cooled tarts in a single layer in a resealable container and freeze. Thaw for 1 to 2 hours. Reheat for 10 minutes in an oven preheated to 225°F.

one 15-ounce package
    refrigerated piecrust
approximately ¼ cup jam

Carrot Cupcakes

🍲 Preparation 15 minutes
🕐 Cook 22 minutes
🧁 Makes 16 cupcakes
☺ Suitable for children under 1
❄ Suitable for freezing:
Baked but un-iced cupcakes
can be frozen for up to 1 month.
Thaw for 2 to 3 hours at room
temperature.

1½ cups self-rising flour
½ teaspoon baking soda
1 teaspoon pumpkin pie spice
a pinch of salt
12 tablespoons (1½ sticks)
    butter, softened
¾ cup (packed) plus
    2 tablespoons light
    brown sugar
3 eggs, beaten
½ teaspoon vanilla extract
2 tablespoons sour cream or
    Greek-style yogurt
1¼ cups grated carrots
⅔ cup raisins

For the icing
1⅓ cups confectioners' sugar
¼ cup maple syrup
¾ teaspoon water
¼ cup chopped pecans, to
    decorate (optional)
marzipan carrots, to
    decorate (optional)

Making cupcakes gives toddlers a more manageable "personal" cake than the traditional large, sliced carrot cake. You could also bake these in ring molds on a baking sheet so that they look like mini carrot cakes with a swirl of icing on top.

Preheat the oven to 375°F. Line two standard muffin pans with 16 paper cases.

Sift together the flour, baking soda, pumpkin pie spice, and salt, and set aside. Beat the butter and sugar in a large bowl until fluffy. Add the eggs, vanilla, sour cream, and dry ingredients, and beat until just combined. Fold in the carrots and raisins.

Spoon the cake batter into the prepared muffin pans, filling each paper case around three-quarters full (an ice cream scoop is good for this). Bake for 18 to 22 minutes, until a toothpick inserted into the centers of the cupcakes comes out clean. Let cool for 5 minutes in the pans, then transfer to a wire rack to cool completely.

To make the icing, put the confectioners' sugar in a bowl and stir in the maple syrup. Add the water, a few drops at a time, to make an icing that will thickly coat the back of a spoon. Spread on the cupcakes and sprinkle with the pecans and top with marzipan carrots, if using.

The iced cupcakes will keep in an airtight container for 3 to 4 days.

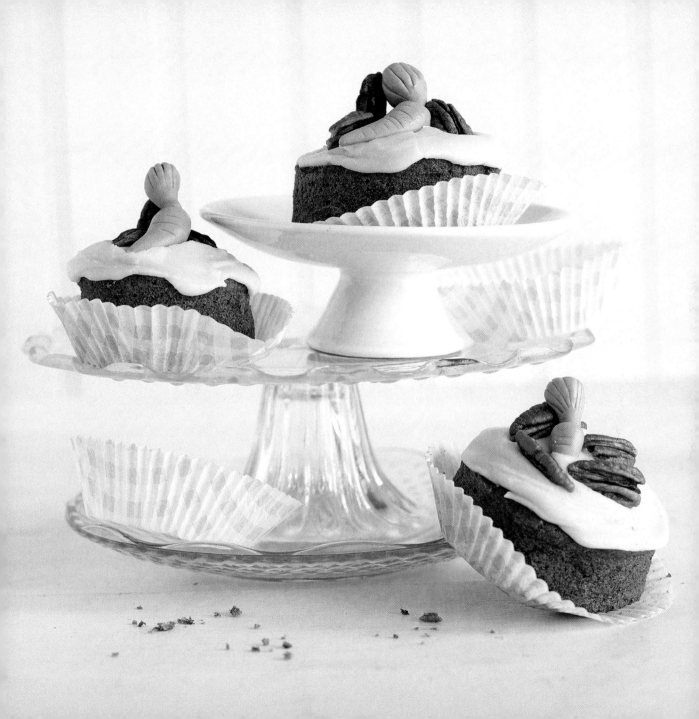

Ice Pops

Fruity ice pops are a great finger food, and one I often recommend to parents whose kids refuse to eat fruit—children can be fooled by a frozen "treat"! The high level of fruit makes these slightly soft, like a sorbet on a stick, so for teething babies it is best to add an extra ⅓ cup water to the orange juice, which will make the pops icier and better for sore gums (the recipe will make about 2½ cups with the extra water).

🍲 Preparation 10 minutes, plus cooling and freezing
🕐 Cook 15 minutes
🍳 Makes about 2¼ cups
☺ Suitable for children under 1

1 medium apple, peeled, cored, and chopped
1 ripe medium pear, peeled, cored, and chopped
⅔ cup chopped dried apricots
½ cup water
2 tablespoons sugar
½ cup fresh orange juice

Apple, Pear & Apricot Ice Pops

Put the apple, pear, apricots, and water in a medium saucepan. Add half of the sugar and put over medium heat. Bring to a simmer, then cover and cook for around 15 minutes, until the fruit is soft. Stir occasionally and add a little extra water if the fruit is looking too dry.

Transfer the cooked fruit to a blender and allow to cool slightly. Add the orange juice and blend until smooth—take care when blending hot liquids. Taste the fruit puree—it should be fairly sweet (and will taste much less sweet when frozen)—and add the remaining sugar, if necessary.

Let cool to room temperature, then pour into ice pop molds and freeze overnight. Best used within 1 month. The puree is also delicious swirled into plain yogurt.

Apple & Mixed Berry Ice Pops

Berries and apples go well together in a fruit crisp and are also perfect partners in an ice pop.

Peel, core, and dice the apples and put them in a medium saucepan with the berries and water. Heat gently until the berries have released some juice, then bring up to a boil and simmer for 5 to 7 minutes, until the apples are soft.

Remove from the heat and stir in the sugar until dissolved. Taste the fruit and add a little more sugar if it is too sharp (this will depend on how ripe the berries are). Puree the fruit and strain to remove the seeds. Let cool, then pour into ice pop molds and freeze overnight. Best used within 1 month.

Preparation 5 minutes, plus cooling and freezing
Cook 7 minutes
Makes 1²/₃ cups
Suitable for children under 1

2 medium apples (I use Fuji)
1 pound mixed berries (e.g., strawberries, blackberries, raspberries, black currants), fresh or frozen
2 tablespoons water
heaping ¹/₃ cup sugar

Mango, Pineapple & Orange Ice Pops

A fun way to use up a slightly overripe mango, these pops can give a little burst of tropical sunshine in winter months.

Put all of the ingredients in a blender and whiz until smooth. If your mango isn't very sweet, then you may need to add an extra tablespoonful of sugar. Pour into ice pop molds and freeze overnight. Best used within 1 month.

Preparation 5 minutes, plus freezing
Makes just over 1 cup
Suitable for children under 1

1 small very ripe mango, peeled, pitted, and diced
one 8-ounce can crushed pineapple, well drained (use pineapple cubes if you can't find crushed)
3 tablespoons fresh orange juice (from a carton is also fine)
¹/₄ cup sugar

"Traffic Light" Fruit Skewers with Creamy Caramel Dip

🍲 Preparation 10 minutes
🍥 Makes 8 skewers, 4 portions
❄ Not suitable for freezing

¼ Galia or other green melon, seeded
½ large mango, peeled, or approximately 5 ounces cut mango
8 medium strawberries, hulled

For the creamy caramel dip
¼ cup dulce de leche
4 teaspoons heavy cream

You will also need 8 plastic or wooden skewers

The red, yellow, and green of these fruits make for an attractive presentation that will appeal to children, but you can use any combination of fruits that your child particularly enjoys.

Remove the rind from the melon and cut 8 cubes, each approximately 1 inch. Cut the mango into 8 similar-size cubes. Thread one cube of melon onto each skewer, followed by a cube of mango and a strawberry.

Mix together the dulce de leche and cream to make the dip, and spoon into small bowls. Serve with the fruit skewers.

Lemon Yogurt Dip Variation
For a tasty alternative dip that is easy to prepare, mix ⅓ cup thick Greek-style yogurt with 2 teaspoons milk, 2 teaspoons confectioners' sugar, and 2 tablespoons lemon curd.

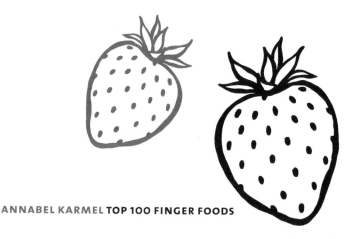

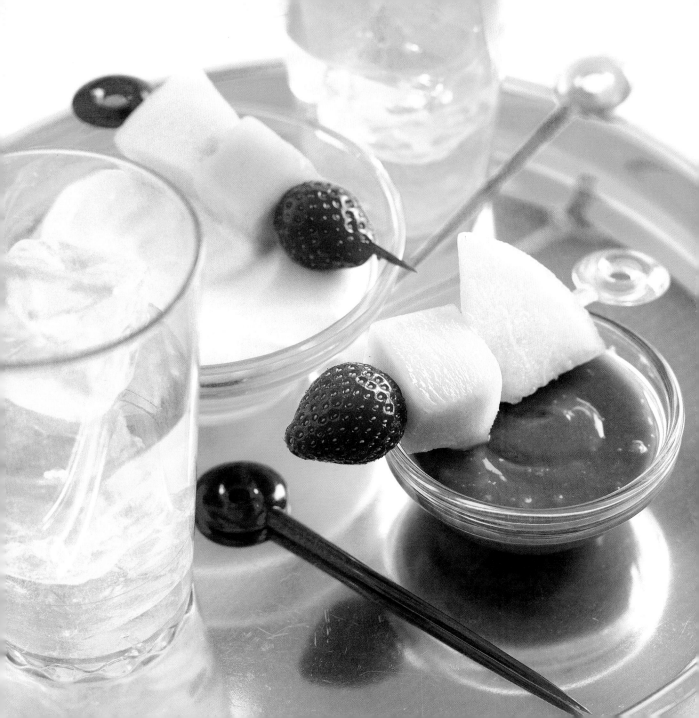

Index

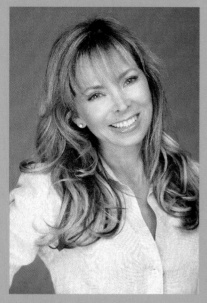

Annabel Karmel is a leading author on cooking for children. After the tragic loss of her first child, who died of a rare viral disease at just three months, she wrote her first book, *The Healthy Baby Meal Planner*, which is now an international bestseller. Annabel has written sixteen more bestselling books on feeding children, including *100 Top Baby Purees, Favorite Family Meals, Complete Party Planner, Lunch Boxes and Snacks,* and *The Fussy Eaters' Recipe Book.* The mother of three, she is an expert at creating tasty and nutritious meals that children like to eat without the need for parents to spend hours in the kitchen. Annabel writes regularly for national newspapers and is a familiar face on British television as an expert on children's nutritional issues.

In the UK, Annabel has her own line of foods in supermarkets based on her popular recipes for children. She has a line called Make It Easy for preparing and storing baby food, and produces cooking sets for children to have fun in the kitchen and learn to cook. She was awarded an MBE (Member of the British Empire) by the Queen in 2006 for her work in the field of child nutrition.

Annabel travels frequently to the United States. She has appeared on many TV programs, including *Live with Regis and Kelly,* the *Today* show, *The View,* and *The CBS Early Show.* She is also a regular on Martha Stewart Living Radio.

For more recipes and advice, please visit www.annabelkarmel.com, or for videos of Annabel's recipes, go to www.annabelkarmel.tv.

Acknowledgments

My children, Nicholas, Lara, and Scarlett, who now don't remember how to use a knife and fork. Caroline Brewster, Marina Magpoc, and Letty Catada for fun times in the kitchen assisting me in testing the recipes for the book. Seiko Hatfield, my wonderful food stylist. Dave King for his magical photography and styling. Jo Harris for the props. Tripp Trapp for the high chairs. My mother, Evelyn Etkind, for her endless support. Thanks to the team at Atria: Judith Curr, Greer Hendricks, Sarah Cantin, Sybil Pincus, Suzanne Fass, Annette Corkey, Judy Eda, Kathleen Schmidt, Christine Saunders, and Chris Lloreda.

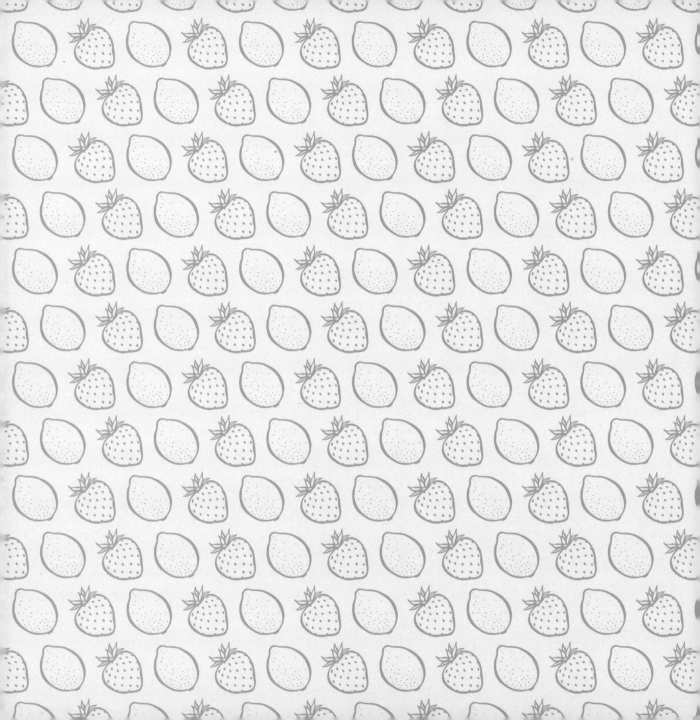